Surviving a Viral Pandemic

SURVIVING A VIRAL PANDEMIC

Through the Lens of a Naturopathic Medical Doctor

HEATHER L. HERINGTON, NMD, DHANP
With contributions by Alec Pekler, NMD and others as noted

ISBN 978-1-7356308-0-9

"Only a crisis - actual or perceived - produces real change. When that crisis occurs, the actions that are taken depend on the ideas that are lying around. That, I believe, is our basic function: to develop alternatives to existing policies, to keep them alive and available until the politically impossible becomes politically inevitable."

Milton Friedman

"There is no mortal whom sorrow and disease do not touch."

Euripides Greek playwright, b.485 BCE

"The horror of a deadly virus being brought into America from overseas reminded me to wish you a Happy Columbus Day."

Anonymous

To my grandchildren and all children: may you keep healthy and happy in harmony with nature.

TABLE OF CONTENTS

PREFACE

Our world is changing fast. With disruptions of food for many, massive economic setbacks as well as disturbances in social connections, our lives are being altered in profound ways. This global pandemic makes one thing abundantly clear: your health needs to be a priority. We no longer have the luxury of postponing it. It's not just someday, but right now.

We live in an era where a highly industrialized agriculture with modernized farming and an unhealthy food industry, together with radiation and environmental toxicities, have resulted in a progressive deterioration of our physical and mental wellbeing.

And that is why the timing of *Surviving A Viral Pandemic* could not be more perfect. And it is also why it is my wish for this book to reach all corners of the world and into the hands of the decision makers and medical authorities that lead the fight against this global pandemic.

During this crisis, the media has made us aware of our mortality like never before. We are bombarded by alarming statistics of death rates and news on how bad things can get. We hear the statistics about how the majority of those losing their lives are suffering from chronic health conditions and comorbidities. And yet, so many of these sources fail to point out that this particular virus is no different than any other in taking people's lives with underlying conditions. People with heart disease, obesity, asthma, autoimmune disease, and type 2 diabetes have always been more vulnerable to sickness and viruses like COVID-19.

Moreover, those in charge of conveying the true facts ignore the startling data confirmed by the Center for Disease Control (CDC) that only 6% of reported deaths were caused by COVID-19 itself; the remaining 94% of patients averaged 2.6 additional conditions. (July 2020).

Let us have a closer look at the types of diseases attributed to this segment of our population:

- According to the CDC, as of 2018, 34.2 million in the US were diagnosed with diabetes-that is 10.5% of the US population. Also, according to the CDC, from 1999–2000 through 2017–2018, the prevalence of obesity increased from 30.5% to 42.4%.

- CDC data also indicates that one person dies every 37 seconds in the United States from cardiovascular disease. About 647,000 Americans die from heart disease each year—that is 1 in every 4 deaths. (2019)
- On the media frontline, the *American Journal of Medicine* reported in 2020 that cancer is the second leading cause of death in the United States, with researchers from the American Cancer Society predicting the disease will affect more than 1.7 million people and cause 600,000 deaths this year.
- Also as stated by the CDC, more than 67,000 people died from drug overdoses in 2018, making it a leading cause of injury-related death in the United States. Of those deaths, almost 70% involved a prescription or illicit opioid. (2019)
- The National Institute of Mental Health, NIH, in 2017 estimated 2.3 million adolescents aged 12 to 17 in the United States had at least one major depressive episode with severe impairment. This number represented 9.4% of the U.S. population aged 12 to 17.
- From the same authority, about 1 in 6 (17%) children aged 3-17 years were diagnosed with a developmental disability, as reported by parents, during a study period of 2009-2017. These included autism, attention-deficit/hyperactivity disorder, blindness, and cerebral palsy, among others.

Putting aside America's dysfunctional health care system, which is really a sick care system, we need to investigate why so many of us are affected, or I should say infected, by such a wide variety of crippling and dangerous pathologies.

Not surprisingly, at least in the eyes of the natural health care practitioner, the modern diet tops the list as the driving force behind epidemic rates of known risk factors for COVID-19 hospitalization and deaths. We live in a toxic consumer culture where junk food companies spend billions on advertising their addictive products while failing to allot a portion of their record earnings towards improving the quality of their ingredients. The stress of environmental contaminants comes in a close second and with most doctors sadly untrained in nutrition or toxicology, no one of authority seems to understand this, or give a damn.

If there has ever been a time our populace needs to be informed of a natural approach to health care by maintaining and reinforcing our body's own immune system, it's right now. Natural medicine providers have known for years that all these chronic conditions are preventable or curable. My colleague and friend, Dr. Heather Herington, can provide the stepping-stones to your new lifestyle, simple actionable steps with daily routines that will help your body protect and heal itself and therefore more easily able to stave off a pathogenic virus.

The stakes are rising exponentially. Every day there's a new story, a new headline detailing statistics of the alarming numbers of those infected and toll this global pandemic is imposing on the lives of so many. Yet, the so-called medical experts, and those public figures on the frontline, have never once offered guidance on how to boost the immune system before a viable vaccine, if there is such a thing, becomes available.

And this is why I am so passionate about this book and why I believe reading it will shed light on so many questions and uncertainties about viruses and our inherent defense system. We never hear on the news how it, our immune system, is perfectly capable of repelling the invader if we take responsibility to educate ourselves on preventive and treatment tools.

Dr. Herington has dedicated her life to helping patients achieve optimal health and overcome many health issues. Her years of hands on clinical experience, in addition to her wealth of knowledge as a naturopathic medical doctor and her mastery of the science of Homeopathy, gives her the expertise that can guide and serve us during this viral pandemic.

Let us together embark on this journey of *Surviving a Viral Pandemic.*

Dr. Atousa Mahdavi, D.C., AHP., B.C.I.M., Yogi
Los Angeles, CA
July 31, 2020

CAUTIONS

Seek emergency medical care immediately for any of the following:

- if there is any blood involved
- trouble breathing
- persistent pain or pressure in the chest
- new confusion
- inability to wake or stay awake
- bluish lips or face
- difficulty walking or speaking
- refusing to drink
- high fever
- severe sore throat
- cough with heavy green mucus production

If you are worried, get tested for SARS-CoV-2 (COVID-19). Because there are many false positive and false negative results, having the more reliable antibody test is recommended.

This book contains in depth information for prevention and home treatment of a viral infection. It can assist you in building resistance, to help your immune system fight off a virus or shorten the intensity and the duration of a viral attack. Additionally, it can help those with a post viral syndrome as in "never well since a viral infection." You can use it to treat the usual "flu" we encounter yearly or now with the novel coronavirus or another virus, even a super influenza virus.

This book is NOT meant to treat a virus like Ebola or that is communicable like HIV/AIDS through bodily secretions.

You can skip the science and philosophy and go straight to protocols but it would be ideal to use the book as a learning tool before a viral infection—similar to the one we are now facing in the spring and summer of 2020—becomes a devastating global event while you still have time to make changes. Learn how to prevent and cure illness through homeopathic and botanical medicine, hydrotherapy, and foods. These treatments can make all the difference.

Prevention is the first step. Do what you can to heal pre-existing chronic conditions before a crisis, with a licensed naturopathic medical doctor or integrated health professional, as having any of these will worsen your ability to withstand a severely mutated and dangerous virus.

1. Heart Conditions or Disease of any kind
2. Lung Conditions or Disease including Asthma
3. Auto-Immune Disease
4. Food or Environmental Allergies
5. Drug and Alcohol Addiction
6. Smoking (although natural tobacco may inhibit the virus)
7. Gastro-intestinal impairments

Keep in mind one reason people like to pop pills is that you simply need to swallow at the direction of a prescription. If you are going to embark on keeping yourself and your family well with natural medicine you will not only have to think but act, possibly in a crisis. It will take focus, understanding and learning. In other words, it will take work.

Be prepared.

INTRODUCTION

Coughing, so dry, so exhaustingly dry. So hot there is a shimmer of sweat. All over. Then chills. Back to hot. Muscles ache. Eyes...the light hurts, they will not stay open. Such fatigue. Deep bone pain where the immune system is revving up the acute attack to get rid of the intruder. More coughing, nothing coming, so dry. No taste. No smell. Nausea. Bowels getting looser. Coming out the other end too…

Whispers and grunts of "Close the curtains!" "A cold drink..." "Tea, really hot." "Just water, please." "Leave me alone." "Another blanket." "Get this sheet off of me!" "Should we go to the hospital?" "I'm not going to the hospital."

Clearly being sick sucks. Whether it's only a cold with a runny nose and mild sore throat or a seasonal flu that wipes us out for weeks after the critter is long gone or now the possibility of a lethal virus that leaked out of a ruined habitat, lurking, ready to leap masked people and tall buildings to hijack your cells.

But what to do? How not to get symptoms or, if diagnosed with a virus like influenza or SARS-CoV-2, what steps can be taken to get better without the dreaded pneumonia staking its claim on your lungs as if you are a new frontier to be owned.

This book was originally written to be prepared for the possibility of an influenza epidemic akin to the so-called 1918 "Spanish" flu. However, before it could be published the COVID-19 crisis exploded into our lives. It now includes relevant research regarding SARS-CoV-2, the virus responsible for COVID-19 (short for coronavirus disease 19) during spring 2020 and will be updated as needed. The general approach to boosting the immune system remains similar.

This is not simply a treatment book that includes the reasons why and what of a recommendation. It also has a historical thread, a narrative to inform readers of why we are in this confusing, deadly time with no mention of natural medicine to help right a virus's wrong. The *tolle causam* (Latin for find the cause) of damaged medical history in the 20th-21st centuries lies in the Flexner Report of 1910 with the robber barons, Rockefeller and Carnegie, hoping to direct us away from nature's offerings and into what they saw as the "science" of medicine. This quickly shortchanged naturopathic medicine and homeopathic medicine, and other systems such as chiropractic, traditional osteopathy, Traditional Chinese Medicine, indigenous medicine that have a firm root in *Vis Medicatrix Naturae,* the healing power of nature.

This historical trauma, that shut down not only "alternative" schools of medicine but women's and black medical schools, and ignored traditional wisdom, has caused the world much *tsouris* (Yiddish for suffering.) The slashing of this knowledge from the stage of possibility is what is missing from the conversation. There are so many ways to reduce suffering, attenuate symptoms, squish the virus like a bug, and most importantly circumvent any chance of deaths due to a viral infection, whether seasonal, or in an epidemic or pandemic. Therefore, those who put their faith solely in mainstream medicine are at a severe disadvantage in a crisis such as we are going through at this time.

Although modern research has been slow to prove efficacy of homeopathy in epidemics or the benefit of foods, plants, water and thought, the reality is natural medicines have had hundreds or thousands of years of trial and error to show us how they can stimulate our vital force and propel our immune system to top shape.

Of course, there are some viruses that are so vicious, like HIV or Ebola, making lab made antivirals extremely welcome to ward them off, but with influenza and SARS-CoV-2 it is not difficult, if we are prepared.

Scientists predicted a pandemic for years although I do not think COVID-19 is the big one. The toll is abominable and continues to rise in the United States and across the world, yet it bears no comparison to the Great Flu of 1918. Of course, that over 500,000 beautiful souls have departed the world is a tragedy from many angles, but it is far, far less than 1918 when up to 50 million people died. This may be Gaia (Mother Earth) giving us a warm-up drill and admonitions. Either way, this is not some out-of-the-blue event we have no control over.

In naturopathic medicine, we hold onto several adages as we make our way to diagnosis and treatment. Finding the cause (*tolle causam*) is a major one. In the case of a pathogenic virus, we see rooted in the stress placed on human health by the progressive destruction of the natural realm we draw on as healers. Deforestation, lack of habitat for wild animals, neglectful animal husbandry, poor nutritional status for humans, pollution—toxic soil, water and air—coupled with mainstream (aka allopathic, conventional) medicine's shameful record of pushing a pill for every disease are all contributors to the dreadful state of health in the American population. These factors are poisoning our environment and ruining our health, possibly for generations. And although this book sticks to health, it's hard to ignore how this pandemic has been mishandled politically, resulting in an economic maelstrom, caused by our inability to work or trust our health-care system, which for too many Americans and for too long, has only cared for those who can afford to be cared for, albeit, at times, improperly. And not to mention how racism and sexism affect our wellbeing.

This is not our first experience in this decade with a health crisis that has had medical personnel scrambling to know what to do. Think back to the summer of 2014 and the sudden emergence of the Ebola virus on the global stage. Nothing for sure was the only constant. Antiviral drugs were not having much luck, sometimes iso-therapy, taking a survivor's blood to boost a sick person, worked, but it was in extremely short supply. It was all a long shot. Experimental every way you looked, watched.

Only one television show I know attempted to discuss the possibility of a deadly global pandemic before the COVID-19 event. The Big Picture with actor/activist Kal Penn offered great visuals, diagrams, and ideas about the various possibilities of an emerging virus. He mentioned Ebola, resident of Africa; Hantavirus, from mouse feces in the Yosemites, California; and Enterovirus D-68, a virus that swooped through the Midwest in the summer of 2014—comes in through the gut, no one died, even as children with asthma were hardest hit. Penn also mentioned the 1918 influenza, highlighting the fact ye olde influenza would become a newer, glossier version, a million times more deadly. And being a resident of North America already it does not have to zoom in on an airplane like Ebola; it just has to mutate, something it does at a very fast clip.

Unfortunately, the smart and hip Penn relied on allopathic or conventional medicine—the system of medicine that has gotten all the press and respect (some warranted, some not) for the last seventy-five years. And strangely, no one else in the media helped prepare for the possibility of using the wide array of natural medicine available either. Instead, as flu season approached, we were told simply to rest in bed, wash our hands (with toxic substances), and get a flu shot. Maybe some radical MD encouraged their patients to take Vitamin C or elderberry but that was a rarity. And no doctor I've encountered mentioned a virus mutating so severely it could be a worldwide tragedy.

On October 18, 2019 Johns Hopkins University ran a simulation of a possible pandemic. It was a disaster, it admitted, according to Ed Cara in his article *We're Not Ready for the Next Pandemic.*[1]

And then it happened. So quickly.

SARS-CoV-2 landed in North America. As the novel coronavirus took center stage quarantines emptied out streets all over the world. People panicked not just by hoarding toilet paper but wondering how they would support themselves and their families. Testing was and still is a fiasco. People with underlying conditions and the elderly in nursing homes began to succumb in large numbers, putting hospitals in fear of overload and for our sick care system in impending paralysis. Even doctors and nurses were dying.

Those of us lucky enough to hide out at home were looking at four walls, digging into old projects or many, stricken with fear, could only watch the news, however devastating and demoralizing. We were standing in line at grocery stores with bandit feeling masks covering our faces and expressions. We would not be going out for dinner although some places had Pick Up and some delivered to doors that wouldn't be opened until the delivery person had left. As a naturopathic medical doctor for over thirty years, I wanted to shout to my neighbors, "There's so much more than hand washing and staying six feet apart to stay healthy!"

Trained as primary care physicians we are experts in Clinical Nutrition, Botanical and Homeopathic medicine, Hydrotherapy, Counseling, all geared to boost the immune system. We have been treating patients for as long as allopaths until the Flexner Report of 1910 put a kibosh on a natural approach to healthcare, failing to understand *Vis Medicatrix Naturae,* the healing power of nature.

Why, with so many extraordinary technological advances, is the best advice to a patient facing a potentially deadly infection merely a thorough hand washing and social distancing?

The answer lies in the fact that our health care is a sick care system, failing to meet our medical needs in the 21st century. I believe in a full spectrum of health care, one that starts with prevention and extends all the way to emergency care. But, to be honest, the dominance of allopathic medicine is why we are where we are. The reigning system is a panic-driven approach as witnessed by attempts to save lives with ventilators while natural medicine on the other hand, and this, in part, explains its unpopularity, works over the long run by first focusing on preventive care rather than waiting for treatment, which in many cases, will sadly be too late. Its time people took an active role in their health, sharing evidence-based scientific knowledge and techniques that have been time-tested through the ages.

Another word to those who think conventional medicine has the answers through vaccines and antivirals. Let me quote Marcia Angell MD from her book, *The Truth About the Drug Companies: How They Deceive Us and What to Do About It*: "It is simply no longer possible to believe much of the clinical research that is published, or to rely on the judgment of trusted physicians or authoritative medical guidelines. I take no pleasure in this conclusion, which I reached slowly and reluctantly over my two decades as an editor of The New England Journal of Medicine."

A few years ago, I sat down to write everything I knew about treating the common flu with naturopathic medicine, what could be extrapolated for an influenza epidemic, or almost any viral epidemic. I began with the theory that conventional medicine works by directly attacking the pathogen, in contrast to the natural approach of building the body's or host response to attack the germ. I read stories from other epidemics, what worked, what did not. I knew people needed to understand the role and benefit of fever and detoxification in acute illness, that aspirin and other fever suppressants can have deadly consequences. Instead of reaching for a drug for every ache or pain we needed to understand that our immune system is an exquisitely orchestrated series of steps. Fresh from writing his Board exams I brought on a new naturopathic grad, Dr. Alec Pekler, who also has a master's in environmental toxicology, for his expertise in optimizing health.

I am aware of the public's disregard for what natural medicine can do but this is 2020. The Flexner Report of 1910 has society gasping for air with its monumental shortsightedness!

To heighten the tension for the moment, viruses that use single stranded RNA instead of the more stable, double stranded DNA as their executive function, are the ones to be concerned about. SARS-

CoV-2, like the influenza virus (second in mutability only to the AIDS virus[2]) is single stranded, a quick-change artist making it next to impossible to determine the correct genome for a vaccine. From a natural medicine perspective, what more do we need to know?

First, we have learned so much more about our immune systems in the last one hundred years. And we have learned what worked in other epidemics. Homeopathy has a proven track record that will be discussed. The plant world first known by indigenous peoples has so much to offer, even with North American research on medicinal plants so slow. Nutrition with vitamins and minerals and other intermediary metabolites (nutraceuticals) saves lives. All of these we can learn to use both to prevent and to treat.

It could feel disheartening to be so brushed aside in terms of knowledge and experience but years ago I took heart from two very special women. One, a tiny yet mighty woman, Marie-Henriette LeJeune, a legendary pioneer who 200 years earlier had lived near my homestead in Cape Breton Island, Nova Scotia. With ancestors both French and Mi'kmaq, Granny Ross, as she was affectionately called, was a midwife, a healer who had a great sense of community and a great love for taking care of people.

Bringing a vial of smallpox serum (and a sharp knife) from France in 1784, LeJeune quarantined family and friends for the few weeks it took to help them recover while keeping a musket for protection against bears. She walked long distances, often across snow and ice, to deliver babies and heal the sick, and through her kinship with the Mi'kmaq, would have learned about Indian Pitcher Plant (*Sarracenia purpurea*) who used it in smallpox. According to Herbert Miles, the Assistant Surgeon to the Royal Artillery, during an outbreak of smallpox: "an old squaw going amongst them and treating the cases with an infusion...was so successful as to cure every case."[3]

The other woman dear to my heart was Georgie Sears, mother of twelve whose farm on the edge of the Tantramarre Marsh was down the rutted road from me when I attended Mount Allison University. She was the embodiment of nature's best, transmitting her love and curiosity of life to all she met. She appreciated my burgeoning interest in herbal medicine and gifted me a copy of the 1919 *The People's Home Library*, a three-inch wide book written by T.J. Ritter M.D., "graduate of both the allopathic and homeopathic schools, formerly assistant to the chair of the theory and practice and medicine, Michigan State University, Ann Arbor, MI." It was the tome her family turned to for medical, cooking, and veterinary advice.

Georgie would scour the marsh for fuzzy leaves to make Labrador tea, the taste of red ripe cranberries, and the beauty of pink or white Mayflowers all the while telling tales of country life, often lying on bare ground under the din of ducks and roaming white clouds in the midst of grey with me, her clueless city-raised neighbor.

Both women have remained an inspiration to me years after abandoning the eight-sided log cabin up in the highlands of Cape Breton that is likely now to be sheltering a moose or two. I like to think I have heard these two women who depended on nature and their own ingenuity to heal the sick whispering in my ear over the years, urging me on.

The good news is individuals know a lot about health these days for the simple reason America as a nation is so unhealthy. Guts are leaky, livers are overloaded; both increasing the chance of food and environmental allergies and toxins. A lot of people now understand there has been an overuse of antibiotics and other drugs, there is too much sugar and refined carbohydrates eaten, that this has also compromised their immunity. We are concerned about GMOs and are aware that heavy metals and pesticides in our air, water, food and/or cosmetics are sitting on receptor sites meant for minerals. We have known for years soil, other than used in organic farming, is depleted. Some, though not nearly enough of us, question vaccines, are perplexed why Vitamin A—known by the World Health Organization (WHO)—is rarely mentioned in conjunction to measles.[4] Add overstimulation from modern society to the mix and we sense our adrenals are exhausted and get why so many yoga studios have sprouted up. We seek peace wherever we can, unfortunately sometimes in something that can lead to an addiction.

Without a doubt much of the population has become better educated, grown more conscious over the last forty-five years or so. The hippies and the back-to-the-landers who read and listened to Rachel Carson have multiplied. These thoughts are now mainstream. Everything is green, green, green.

Except healthcare.

Because knowing ways to gain health when a healing crisis

occurs does not make it a given. Human nature tells us we may swear we want to do what is natural, what works with the body but then we become afraid and make choices based on our level of fear. Instead of trusting in our body's immune system we rely on what we are told is needed to stay safe, and in too many cases, cover up that initial discomfort with a pill, adhering to a quick-fix from your family doctor. Not being trained to negotiate our body's needs, we revert to our sphere of comfort without understanding the basics of healing.

To be sure, having limited knowledge is not on you. The disturbing fact is there is very little said about boosting the immune system. In Canada, regarding COVID-19, friends say they are encouraged to eat well, to consume vegetables and fruits to gain needed nutrients but in California where I am there is nary a word. The theories and basis of naturopathic medicine[5] are unknown or ignored. Even the excellent Special operations Forces Nutrition Guide, written for Navy Seals, is disregarded, a manual that goes into detail of how to maximize the benefit of food.[6]

It is common knowledge that most people who die from a viral infection do so because they have compromised immune systems before an offending virus enters the nasal passages. They have underlying conditions such as high blood pressure, COPD, diabetes—with the majority being elderly—often from years of a poor diet, no matter how much money they earn or have, and years of ingestion of toxic chemicals as well as chronic dehydration. Or emotional suppression.

The reality is we all have the ability to make better choices: to get to the bottom line of what is healing, what is helpful to our wellbeing.

We cannot deny the many technological advances over the last hundred years. Cleaner cities with better sewage and electricity allowing refrigeration have saved countless lives. Many drugs are lifesaving.

But we went too far. Over prescribing antibiotics in humans and the unregulated use in livestock production has resulted in antibiotic resistant organisms, not to mention possible health consequences. Big Pharma (the pharmaceutical industry) is too concerned with profit margins to be trusted, and many medical doctors are too concerned with malpractice to give you any real alternative to a vaccine or antivirals. The dominant medical profession, whose philosophy is rarely questioned, doesn't trust nature or its medicinal value. It doesn't believe in the healing power of nature, nor has it yet conceded that integrated medicine may have answers to our health care crisis. The emphasis is still on cure at all cost vs. prevention at a fraction of the cost.

And although few know the Latin phrase, *Vis Medicatrix Naturae*—once more with feeling, the healing power of nature—this concept has crept into the public's consciousness in the last twenty or so years. Through necessity many people have discovered natural medicines.

By making better choices based on bona fide research as well as keeping an ear out for anecdotal experience to put to the test, we build our strength, optimize our host response, wrangle a cell-mediated Th1 immune response that allows for elimination/detoxification to make it more difficult for a pathogen to infiltrate our bodies and overwhelm our inner ecosystem.

Prevention, of course, is key. How we react to stress is clearly based on what we eat, how well we sleep, what we think and feel, what our environment offers us, even how deeply we breathe. Every day we need to think about reducing unwanted stress, creating a life that pares away what doesn't serve us. With reflection and knowledge, we increase good habits.

But nothing is guaranteed. We have no idea when any virus will appear or in what form. Even with COVID-19 being the focus, the possibility still looms that the annual influenza virus will throw a curveball, possibly be as devastating as 1918 when symptoms were ghastly with hemorrhages from the nose, mouth and lungs not uncommon.

Exploring a healthcare protocol that we can trust to keep us safe when an unfriendly microorganism invades our system makes the most rational choice. It may all come down to what information you have and what experience has taught you and whom you can rely on. Public Health tells us to wash our hands, cover our mouths and noses, cough into our elbows, stay 12 feet apart and yet, there is so much more we can do, all the while the CDC continues to push a flu shot or if you can wait 12 to 18 months a vaccine for COVID-19. Perhaps there is a passing mention of pharmaceutical antivirals, but in what quantity and accessibility are these being stockpiled? [7]

Generations ago we didn't know not to trust what seemed extraordinary medicine coming after World War II with the advent of antibiotics. But now the dilemma of a system that relies on drugs is coming into question. And it's not just drugs, rather it's drugs for plants like the ubiquitous and pervasive glyphosate and other (so-called by Monsanto "inert") chemicals in the weed killer, Round Up® that are creating real and terrible danger to our genetics, our thyroid glands and more. We have the right to know what we can do proactively for our best health, preventively and in a crisis.

For some, already well-versed in prevention and the role of toxic chemicals, it may be as simple as monitoring hydration and electrolytes. Others can learn more about beneficial foods and supplements, the role of toxic chemicals, botanical medicine, homeopathic medicine, hydrotherapy, as well as meditation, yoga, and visualization. They can do much to engage the little white blood cells roaming our capillaries and lymph just waiting to snap up an invading pathogen.

And it's not just for us but for our community.

When I offered an early draft of this book to my college housemate, Mary Minor ND, then of Alaska, she let me know about the experience of the Yup'ik people, who, to this day, grapple with the consequences of a 1900 influenza and smallpox outbreak in their villages. Again, my head was reeling, my heart hurting. Because although I specialized in treating PTS for three decades, I had never known epidemics had left their mark for over a century.

Larry McMurtry, in his novel *Some Can Whistle,* wrote "...the Incas could lay stones together so skillfully and delicately that the stones could even pass the shock of earthquakes from one to another in such a way that the building they composed wouldn't fall down. Spanish buildings erected over Inca buildings fell down in seconds, but the Inca buildings remained."[8]

This book is about laying stones of knowledge, placing each in a way that has something to benefit our immune system in order to stay healthy or recover more quickly with a potent virus in our midst. To understand that we can find stones, alone and together, that will add to a truly holistic approach to a global tragedy is the purpose of these pages.

Cultivate your knowledge as you expand your definition of what you can do for yourself and your family, the need has never been greater. By learning the basics of natural healing to better withstand a pathogenic virus we up our chances of keeping our family and community well or helping them recover more quickly, physically and psychologically.

Remember the Incas; keep the stones of healing balanced!

It is time for all of us to wake up, to acknowledge that our continued dominance over nature has resulted in quite the pickle.

The good news is we can do something about it.

PART ONE: INFECTIOUS DISEASE

CHAPTER 1: SHAPING HUMAN HISTORY

PATHOGENS

It is said that infectious disease caused by a pathogen, whether a virus that can't be seen with the naked eye, or bacteria, protozoan, fungi or worms, has been the single most important factor in shaping human history. They have affected what we eat, where we live, our cultures, national and global economies and more. Although we don't know the extent this present experience of COVID-19 will add to this we do know it already has affected us not just in the tragic loss of life from the virus and suicide from loneliness but in economic insecurity, and a questionable path forward.

From 1348-1350 in Europe, Black Death aka the bubonic plague, killed two-thirds of the population and, with no cure in sight, or means of obtaining an income, city dwellers hastily retreated to rural life.

In 1623, the Pope, ten of his cardinals and hundreds of aides died when mosquitoes rose up from Rome's marshes and spread malaria but in this case a cure, quinine, from the bark of the cinchona bark, was discovered, becoming more valuable than gold.

We also know that indigenous cultures, and not just in North America, were decimated in numbers along with their cultural identity that continues to be felt to this day due to an invisible microbe. A little-known fact, some peoples like the Taino in Hispaniola, an extraordinary culture of invention and pharmacy, were on the verge of extinction by the early 1500s thanks to Columbus.

Historically, a pathogenic germ, its source unknown, has elicited sheer terror among the human population. Today seems no different. The atmosphere surrounding this ranges from trepidation to outright panic due to our inability to understand a virus and its capabilities.

We have studied the first swine flu of 1918 (we didn't know it was a virus until the discovery of the electron microscope in the 1930s) and we will study SARS-CoV-2, commonly known as COVID-19.

Public sanitation and personal hygiene has had a lot to do with the reduction of morbidity and mortality of infectious disease.[1] We grasp the role of sanitation, crowded conditions, environmental toxins and nutritional status yet still there is tremendous insecurity around these invisible-to-the-eye little buggers, and that lies in the fact we have not reached a level of understanding of what actually makes us sick and how to restore health. We haven't understood the need for a healthy, diverse gut microbiome or the necessary element of elimination in the cycle of healing to fight off an infectious disease.

In total, there have been 400 emerging, or new infectious diseases since the beginning of World War 2 with 60% of these being zoonotic, meaning they come from animals.[2] This crossover is an old trick. Measles originated from the domestication of livestock a long, long time ago. The source for the Ebola virus is bats as seems to be SARS 1 (severe acute respiratory syndrome), and SARS-CoV-2 (COVID-19) and MERS (middle east respiratory syndrome) while HIV comes from monkeys and influenza from birds and pigs or simply a change or deletion in an amino acid sequence. In the end, it may all come down to deforestation and crowded conditions.

We have so much to learn to keep in balance with nature; unfortunately, this may seem barbaric to certain people who believe dominance of nature is the only way out of the mess we have created. What really interests me is how people, without being guided by government but their own ingenuity, have dealt with a deadly disease.

Consider smallpox, the scourge across Europe and Asia for centuries that killed 300-500 million people including 90% of the indigenous population of North, Central and South America.[3] Originally communicated by rodents, smallpox was described in Indian texts as early as 1500 BCE, and found on an Egyptian mummy in 1145 BCE. It hit Japan in 735-737 CE, killing one-third of the population.

It roamed Africa, the Middle and Far East for thousands of years and by the 16th century was blowing across Europe like an evil wind. Becoming the leading cause of death in the 18th century, it killed Chief Sitting Bull, Aztec Chief Cuitlåhuac, the Inca ruler Huayna Capac and 80% of the First Nations through exposure to often intentionally contaminated blankets.

To counter this often deadly and disfiguring disease, variolation (from the Latin word for smallpox, *Variola*) was practiced. Using ground up scabs and fluid from pustules either blown up a person's nose (Chinese 1000 BCE) or scratched into the skin with a lancet or bifurcated points (Middle East, Africa, Nova Scotia), while another technique, used in late 1700s Sudan, is similar to the goal of chicken pox parties today. A mother would barter with the mother of an infected child and after agreeing on a price per pustule, tie a cloth around the child's arm and return home to tie it around their own child's arm. Although there was still risk of death, it was much less, .5 to 2 % compared to 30 to 35% if the disease itself was contracted.[3]

EVOLUTION OF KNOWLEDGE OF THE UNSEEN

A few centuries ago, when no one had a clue what a virus or other pathogen was, what it could do or what it looked like, the term "spontaneous generation" arose. This common belief held that life could arise from non-life or inorganic material. For example, people assumed that maggots simply appeared on rotting meat. The idea was trashed in 1668 when the Italian physician Francesco Redi proved that maggots did not just spontaneously appear. They came, in fact, from flies that had laid tiny eggs on the rotting meat. The maggots were simply the intermediary or larval stage in the cycle of a fly.

This discovery occurred about the same time as Dutch lens-maker Antonie van Leewenhoek's (1632-1723) first visualization of microbes (a general term that covers all microscopic organisms, healthy or unhealthy) through a primitive microscope. He didn't know exactly what he was looking at but as it turned out it was a bacterium, not the much, much smaller entity of a virus.

The game was on, if slowly, to discover the cause of people falling ill. Many theories crept in and it was well over a century later that Louis Pasteur (1822-95) in Paris and Robert Koch (1843-1910) in Berlin established germs as the cause of infectious diseases.[4]

Pasteur too had dispelled the concept of "spontaneous generation," by demonstrating the existence of airborne microscopic "germs" while Koch isolated the first bacterium, *Bacillus anthracis.*

Richard Pfeiffer, a scientist in Germany who, in 1892, described rod-shaped bacilli (bacteria) and for years this was the accepted culprit in flu. But when he couldn't replicate it in experimental animals' bacteriology methods, more scientists disagreed and continued to create vaccines from other bacteria.[5]

Over time, and to make a longer story shorter there remained a group of infectious diseases that could not be isolated to a causative organism. These microbes were called "filterable agents" in light of the fact they were getting through the material the scientists used to trap bacteria and other pathogens. They decided these "filterable agents" must be extremely small but considered them, simply, tiny bacteria.

Then, in 1898, Martinus Beijerinck, a microbiology teacher at an agricultural school in Holland coined the word "virus."

Building on Adolf Mayer's work in Holland and later Dmitry Ivanovsky in Russia, Beijerinck repeated filter experiments (on plants, how it was normally done) and showed that the "filterable agent" they hoped to isolate grew in dividing cells and manifested its strength each time it infected a plant. He deemed the agent a living microbe and gave it the name "virus" from the Latin word for poisonous venom or slimy fluid.

But even by the early 1900s the nature of a virus remained a mystery, other than that it was infectious and needed living cells as a host to propagate.

In 1918, the virus that caused the so-called "Spanish" Flu that killed millions was still invisible. It wasn't until the 1930s when German engineer Max Knoll and physicist Ernst Ruska invented the electron microscope that viruses could finally be visualized. (By accelerating electrons and relying on the reality of a corresponding wave of any given particle, these scientists, standing on the backs of many, defeated the limitation of what could be seen by visible light.)

Between 1935-1940 the American biochemist Wendell Stanley, working with the tobacco mosaic virus, proved that viruses contain protein. Then two English biochemists discovered viruses contain nucleic acids.

In 1953 through the work of James Watson and Francis Crick the genetic spiral of DNA and RNA was uncovered as the brains of any cellular operation, including viruses.

By 1964 molecular biologist Howard Temin proposed that some viruses use RNA, some DNA as their genetic information. (It would take two years before this idea was acknowledged and accepted.)

Approximately twenty years later the proteins of viruses were identified, leading to vaccines, including the yearly one for influenza,[6] and then, more recently, to antiviral drugs. It's no wonder scientists were excited to finally put a face on a virus that had caused such suffering and death and is one reason I believe that technological advances were given a pass. To feel helpless and be unable to offer anything concrete for so long made scientists search for ways to destroy the pathogens, *i.e.* unhealthy microbes that seemed intent on killing humans. No one could have foreseen antibiotic or antiviral resistance or that these tiny things have a use in evolution and that we need to understand their role in a broader ecosystem.

ASSIGNMENT #1

1. Define zoonotic and why this is dangerous. Can you think of ways to avert this?
2. How did H1N1 in 1918 become an emerging virus?
3. What is the name of the virus that leads to the disease, COVID-19 and where did it come from?
4. What have you learned about infectious disease during COVID-19 and what are you doing differently in your life?

CHAPTER 2: VIRUSES

JUST WHAT ARE THEY?

If viruses could speak, they would have a long story to tell. They have been around for two to three billion years, all the way back to when life on Earth consisted of one-celled bacterium. Yet it hasn't even been a hundred years, since the discovery of the electron microscope, that we can see viruses and know they are the cause of disease including yellow fever, chicken pox, smallpox, Ebola, AIDS, the common cold, influenza, SARS, MERS, and SARS-CoV-2 (COVID-19).

Yet the majority of viruses are harmless. They do not infect us negatively. Rather they are essential for evolution. Wolfherd Weidel wrote on the cover of his 1959 book, *Virus*: "Nothing brings us closer to the riddle to life—and to its solution—as viruses." Bernard Dixon in his book, *Power Unseen*, wrote, "A small bacterium weighs one trillionth of a gram and a blue whale 100 million grams. Yet a bacterium can kill a whale." And a virus is oh so much smaller than any bacteria could ever dream of being.

The medicalese or fancy speak for a virus is an obligate intracellular parasite. This means a virus is a parasite that is obligated to use another living thing's cellular apparatus in order to survive. Yet with as much havoc as a virus is capable it is not considered a living substance to most scientists. It cannot replicate on its own, breathe oxygen, can't ingest food or eliminate waste. We can't see them as they float around in the air, or on water, or in food, just waiting to invade a living organism so they can survive. With no reproductive capabilities of their own they have no choice but to link up to one of our host cells, pirating the cell's machinery.

A virus is completely and utterly dependent on another life to survive. It can use our cells and also replicate inside a bacterium, a plant or an animal. They are parasites through and through, hijacking living cells to do their bidding.

VIRAL STRUCTURES

Viruses vary greatly in shape, size, and complexity but they all share two basic structures: the genetic material of a nucleic acid core, either DNA, double stranded genetic material, or RNA (a single strand of genetic string and what an influenza and COVID-19 cell have), and a protein coating that protects this core, called the capsid. An outer envelope—made of lipids and proteins just like a regular cell does—enables the virus to recognize receptor proteins in the host cell's membrane allowing the virus to expand its territory.

What is missing from a virus is the endoplasmic reticulum and ribosome and cytoplasm as you might remember from high school biology class. The virus must force the host cell to become its slave for a day or two until the host bursts open from all the copies being made inside it. But by that time, it is too late for us. The virus has done what it set out to do: replicate itself.

All viruses have their specialty. The host cell they are attracted to may be in your nose (SARS-CoV-2) or another orifice. Their traveling route can be by air (influenza and possibly SARS-CoV-2) or by water or through food. Whatever part of the body and whatever route, the virus pierces the membrane of its new host so it can enter in order to divide and conquer.

Only new viruses, or more accurately, new combinations of older viruses, can destroy us. Over history many have been eradicated or minimized. Even the virus of a common cold could have killed you if you had lived thousands of years ago. As our bodies came to know this virus, our immune system was challenged, over and over, to garner an appropriate response. Once a devastating and terminal viral attack occurred, we finally became "immune" and now the common cold is just an annoyance that leaves our heads stuffed up, our noses running but it does not kill.

The danger of a new virus, known as "emerging," means it will have less chance of being recognized by the immune system. The influenza and COVID-19 viruses are only two of many possible emerging viruses that scientists are concerned about in the 21st century.

Consider Ebola: In 1976 in Zaire, when the Ebola virus first emerged from the jungles of Central Africa, transferred from animal to human, it annihilated 90% of the population since humans had not encountered this viral pattern. Victims died within a week of exposure, not enough time for the host to spread the virus, and they both withered away and died. Or so we thought. Instead, lingering in reservoirs and as previously mentioned, it took forty years for it to make another and more monumental entrance in 2014, again letting loose on previously unexposed populations that have no resistance.

This type of deadly transmission in which people have little protection is no different from the genocidal ability of the smallpox virus (also measles and influenza) regarding the indigenous peoples in North America and the Aztecs in Mexico. Unintentionally, these viruses were brought to the New World by Columbus and Cortés, but later were intentionally used to conquer these people, true genocide in action as with Lord Jeffrey Amherst infecting blankets with smallpox with the Native Americans/First Nations.

Another possibility of emerging viruses is that they are escaping from labs due to a lack of safety protocols but in depth coverage is beyond the scope of this book except to say that stewardship and safe ecological practices on our planet and in labs must be strengthened if we are going to minimize the danger of emerging viruses.

INTERACTION WITH THE BODY'S DEFENSE SYSTEM

When a pathogenic virus is on the horizon, your immune system—our body's defense system—begins to take action. The innate immune system, already on the alert for unwanted pathogens, wakes up the adaptive or acquired immune system. White blood cells, mainly natural killer cells and cytotoxic lymphocytes, gobble up or phagocytize the virus. Thankfully, or we would all be dead, these two processes usually kill the virus. But if they do not, the body is forced to replicate a lot of new viruses, causing an infection, making us potentially very sick.

THE FLU VIRUS: A FAMILIAR FOE BECOMING A SUPER FLU

The influenza virus, a member of the Orthomyxoviridae family, is a single stranded, highly mutable RNA virus. Originally attributed to the "influence" of the heavenly bodies, this potentially devastating virus became known as influenza early on in human history.

Transmitted through the air, only 80 to 120 nm in size, the influenza virus produces an upper and lower respiratory infection that inflames and damages the larynx, trachea and bronchi and can lead to a deadly bacterial pneumonia.

Symptoms include fever, nasal and throat congestion, body aches, and possibly a rash. But that can be just the beginning. More violent symptoms, as seen in the 1918 epidemic described below, included profuse nosebleeds and hemoptysis, blood coughed up from the respiratory system. Some chroniclers noted bleeding from the ears, explosive coughing that tore apart abdominal muscles and rib cartilage; also noted were terrible headaches, skin changes including blue around the lips or fingertips signifying cyanosis (lack of oxygen), vomiting, intense body aches, and writhing.[1]

Distinct from Ebola and other viral infections, the influenza virus is right at home in North America and Europe and does not need an airplane to make an appearance. It lives and breeds among us in the annual outbreak of seasonal "flu." This is not a bacterium—with a known structure an antibiotic can kill (until it cannot)—but an RNA virus that continually changes its shape, easily eluding any attempt at a match for a vaccine. A highly mutating pathogen especially when pigs and birds are involved, it is extremely difficult to pin down and eradicate.

And that is the "clear and present" danger we face today.

TYPES

Influenza A virus can infect humans, birds, swine along with seals and horses. Influenza B affects only humans and seals so no crossover concern with regards to avian or swine. Influenza C can infect humans and swine, but it is very rare.

Influenza A and B virus types and their subgroup cause most illness in humans and are the culprits in seasonal flu. The subgroups of A include H1N1 and H3N2 while B has what are called "lineages," classified either Victoria or Yamagata. These have further subgroupings called clades and then sub-clades. (So, you can see how hard it is to exact the correct pattern for the flu vaccine.) Influenza A viruses are the only influenza viruses known to cause an influenza global pandemic.

THE INFLUENZA A VIRUS

Influenza A virus has a nucleic acid core of RNA, ribonucleic acid, and so has a very high rate of mutation, only the HIV virus is higher. It can amount to a million times more than that of a virus with DNA as its core.

Shaped like a corkscrew, it has eight twists, each containing the genetic material and a lipid bilayer with spikes that enable the virus to bind with the host cell. Only two of these are of real concern: hemagglutinin (H or HA) and neuraminidase (N or NI) aka sialidase. Subtypes come from H1-H16 and N1- N9, each drastically different from the other yet share the same function as host receptor-destroying enzymes.

Manipulating the host cell machinery to reproduce, the virus remains attached to the cell's surface by binding between hemagglutinin and sialic acid. Hemagglutinin acts like glue in the binding, fusion, and entry process of the virus into the host cell. Neuraminidase is an enzyme that cleaves sialic acid linkages essential for release of progeny virus from the surface of the cell and can infect other cells. These are highly susceptible to mutation.

Neuraminidase inhibitors include drugs such as Tamiflu® (oseltamivir) and Relenza® (zanamivir). NIs are also in botanicals, although it seems HA is more at play.

THE DANGER OF MUTATION OR ANTIGENIC DRIFT

As discussed earlier, the ability to conjure new strains of itself is what makes the influenza virus so dangerous. It is ever evolving; as a result, the immune system is always trying to catch up, exerting itself with the challenge of confronting the new, mutated virus. Meanwhile the virus travels through the air, circulates within a family, a school, or a community looking for new host cells to infect.

Thus, one might say the virus outwits us at every turn by changing its structure. And when our genetic material, our RNA, is swapped between different viral strains of pigs and ducks, watch out!

The Zimmerman brothers, in their book, *Killer Germs*, call pigs "nature's true mixing bowl for flu viruses" because if a human flu virus replicates inside a pig it can triangulate with an H or N gene from a duck. This is why the 1918 pandemic would ultimately be called the first swine flu.

Saunders and Hastings argue, "...pandemic influenza is in part a consequence of human development, and highlights the importance of considering outbreaks within the context of a shifting global landscape."[2] This sounds like a good topic for discussion that may link developed and undeveloped countries with clean water and food.

SPREADING

It's easy in North America to keep pigs and humans apart but not so easy in countries in Asia where their farming practices rely on polyculture, meaning hens are kept above pigs and feed on their feces. These pig feces then fertilize ponds where ducks swim...well, you get the picture.

What seems to be true as well as frightening is that influenza viruses can thrive in the digestive tract of these critters—pigs and ducks—with no harmful effect on them. So, they don't die off.

It is the proficiency of spreading, the transmission of the viral vector that is often the determining factor in causing a widespread disease.[3] For instance, the H5N1 (bird) flu cannot spread between humans (it first jumped from birds to humans in 1997) but it was a major scare in 2005 (from ducks in Vietnam). Fortunately, this H5N1 is poorly adapted to its human host because of its inability to transmit efficiently. It does not become airborne; it is not therefore transmissible when people sneeze or cough.

A virus' continuing ability to make changes genetically is why there are regular yearly outbreaks of the "flu" and then every decade or so an epidemic of some level of influenza. The past century has seen pandemics from viruses of the H1, H2 and H3 subtypes but not H5 although it is circulating in flocks of birds throughout the world and needs only five mutations in its gene code to possibly become transmissible between humans.[3] If this happens or two different strains of another subtype recombine into a new version of the influenza virus capable of illness in humans, we are in serious trouble.

In fact as of this writing in July 2020, there is a new virus that is genetically descended from H1N1 that has emerged from "the massive pig farm industry in China" due to a pig surveillance program that started after the H1N1 2009 outbreak. This information comes from research in PNAS[4] that announces, "this virus has all the essential hallmarks of a candidate for a pandemic virus."

However, novel influenza strains resulting in a human pandemic have emerged for centuries. Greek writings from 412 BC seem to describe a widespread influenza outbreak although one from Asia (spread by land routes to North Africa, then Europe and North America) in the summer of 1580 is considered the very first influenza pandemic.[2]

PANDEMIC INFLUENZA

Likewise, following the first swine flu, H1N1, of 1918-19 the result of a ménage a trois from a pig and bird to join a human gene[4] became a devastating global affair, we have had several concerning influenza epidemics or pandemics:

Year	Description
1957- 8	from birds, H2N2 "Asian" flu, 1 - 2 million deaths
1968	added genes from wild ducks, H3N2 "Hong Kong" flu, 500,000 to 2 million deaths
1977	"Russian flu" version of H1N1 (an escapee from a Russian lab) 700,000 Russians died
2009-10	another H1N1, Swine Flu Mexico. This is the only one not suspected to have its source in China, up to 575,000 deaths

All subtypes were from viruses of H1, H2, and H3 subtypes (more on this in a bit) not H5 although H5 is circulating in flocks of birds throughout the world and needs only five mutations in its gene code to possibly become transmissible between humans.[3]

THE GREAT FLU OF 1918

The Great Flu of 1918 sums up much of what we need to know about how the medical, cultural, and environmental circumstances can evolve into a pandemic.

One of the most devastating pandemics humankind has ever experienced, influenza struck during the last year of World War I and was erroneously nicknamed the Spanish Flu because all other countries—Britain, France, Canada, the USA and others—but not Spain had a media blackout on coverage of it in order to not give enemies an advantage. It erupted in Fort Riley, Kansas, as men were getting ready to go overseas to fight. Consider this:

It is March 11, 1918. There has been a dust storm that has mixed with burning manure from thousands of army horses and mules that are getting ready to go overseas to battle. There is a haze above the fort and the cook comes down with a bad cold. One hundred men also get sick with a similar presentation to the cook. But then forty-eight soldiers die, attributed to pneumonia. Before you know it 84,000 soldiers ship out to Europe and then 118,000 the next month. Six soldiers die on the ship crossing the Atlantic Ocean. Now Europe is infected with soldiers on both sides beginning to die. By July whatever this is has struck soldiers and civilians in North Africa, Russia, India, China, Japan, the Philippines, as far as New Zealand.[1]

The virus mutates, making it impossible for the immune system to fight back easily and when it arrives back across the Atlantic to the good ol' USA, it becomes a devastating situation. No one has seen anything like this before.

In late August and early September doctors at Chelsea Naval Hospital in Boston are shaken to discover that bloody, foamy liquid is drowning the soldiers' lungs. Three people in nearby Quincy die. The unknown assailant is an airborne virus and at the parade 'A Win the War for Freedom' it ends up spreading the disease to the rest of the population. One thousand people die within a month.

No one knows what to do since they haven't even seen a virus under a microscope because an electron microscope won't be invented for another 20 years!!

The first wave in January 1918 looked like a normal seasonal flu-killing the elderly and the young—but the second was deadly for those 20-40 years old. Lungs filled with fluid with monumental hemorrhaging of infected lung cells, arteries bursting open due to an over-stimulating cytokine storm that then spread to the GI tract, the brain, epithelial cells...everywhere mucous membranes made a connection and increased inflammation. Bleeding erupted from the nose, mouth, GI, even ears.

One doctor wrote that only moments after admission mahogany spots could appear on cheek bones; a few hours later cyanosis (blueness, lack of oxygen) would extend from the ears and spread all over the face. "It's only a matter of hours until death comes, and it is simply a struggle for air until they suffocate."[1]

During this time local governments took measures... people in San Francisco were forced by law to wear masks...elsewhere whole towns were quarantined; public places were closed. In San Diego, a law forced people to wear gauze masks in the street. A government rhyme went like this:

"Obey the laws
And wear the gauze
Protect your jaws
From septic paws."

By November 1918, eight months after it started, the pandemic died down, disappearing as fast as it came on. (Other reports cite summer or Fall 1920.) Perhaps it was the varying in intensity of symptoms although for our purposes it doesn't matter the exact dates. It matters that it disappeared and what we can learn from it.

Historically, the numbers of the infected and the deceased due to the influenza virus differ but 50 million of both categories amounting to one hundred million globally is commonly reported. And what is not refuted is that never has a disease spread so quickly and killed so many in such a short time with doctors and nurses and other health workers as well as morticians being the first casualties. (The only place in the world not affected was the small and isolated island of Marajø in Brazil's Amazon River basin.)

ASSIGNMENT #2

1. What does antigenic drift mean and how does that influence your choices in resisting a virus?
2. What does H and N refer to in an Influenza A virus?
3. What are three things you remember about the Great Flu of 1918?
4. How may that apply to life present day?

CHAPTER 3: OUR IMMUNE SYSTEM

THE DANCE TO KEEP US WELL

Even if it feels initially like too much science, I want you to get a sense of what an immune response is in a viral pandemic. What it can do. In this way we won't feel the rush for a vaccine. We can work with what nature has given us, give it what it needs so it can keep or get us well. Because that's what it's there for: to propel us toward good health.

And if nothing else, read this paragraph: contemplate the work of the white blood cells that swallow pathogens or spray them with noxious chemicals, egged on by cytokines, in step with the lymphatic system that acts as a garbage disposal, that runs alongside the blood vessels, and all the other metabolites. This pretty spiffy defense system is our inherent machinery that ensures us both safety and health, a system we can rely on as long as we supply it what it needs, what this book is ultimately about.

Truly a finely tuned dance, our immune system hums along in the background of every moment of our life. Seeking to protect us from disease through pummeling invading toxins, our inner defense network of cells, tissues and organs work as one. The interplay of the bloodstream, lymphatic system and fixed anatomical structures create a beautifully orchestrated series of steps. By learning friend and foe to this extraordinary response whether through diet, exercise, plants and so on we can enhance or diminish its abilities.

In a viral infection, the most ancient part, the innate immune system, continually looking out for any pathogenic microbe system 24/7, springs into action with the recognition of a potentially harmful microbe and then, when overwhelmed, will harness the relatively more recent adaptive or acquired immune system for further neutralization and elimination. To be honest, what these two systems have is beyond extraordinary; the word "miracle" comes to mind.

Nonspecific defense mechanisms are in play long before a

potentially sickly or deadly virus makes an appearance. And once a microbe does it immediately adds to its repertoire. Epithelial barriers include tight junctions, keratin in skin making it too dry for a virus to attach itself to and sweat with its lowered pH that also inhibits attachment. The linings in our nose, mouth, upper airways, lungs, and GI tract repel the virus while cilia in our lungs move mucus up to the pharynx so the virus can be coughed up.

Natural acids such as fatty acids on the skin, lysosomes in saliva, and hydrochloric acid in the stomach help by changing the pH or breaking down proteins of the virus. Other highly toxic oxygen-derived compounds—superoxide, hypochlorite—HOCL, hydrogen peroxide, hydroxyl and nitrate radicals—lead to respiratory bursts that kill the virus. These are generated by neutrophils and macrophages although neutrophils are short-lived and die in this process, becoming the major component of pus. Research has recently uncovered an innate antiviral pathway that works at the epithelial (skin) surface before interferon gets involved. This pathway is activated to stimulate anti-viral activation-dependent neutrophils.[1] All of this without even mentioning our microbiota—balanced gut flora—that enables a strong terrain (microbiome) that has added to the chances a virus won't take.[2]

THE WHITE BLOOD CELLS (WBCS)

White blood cells (WBCs) are the stars on the immune stage... whoo-whoo! ... emerging from bone marrow and transforming into an assortment of WBCs to offer protection. Activation of innate immune cells through toll-like receptors and the complement system[3] ensure viruses are sought and snagged, and then cleared away by macrophages.

There are two types of macrophages - M1 and M2. M1s produce toxic metabolites (such as nitric oxide) to kill a pathogenic microbe. M2 ingests dead cells, infectious microbes and clears away the debris generated. Charles Mills discovered this polarization before dying in 2017 saying this is more important than the T cell activity in effecting healing. This is ongoing research. What's important to remember is that M2 macrophages are activated by cytokines and glucocorticoids *i.e* cortisol and that elimination, its primary job, is absolutely essential to any healing.

WBCs, in the first line of defense, also include mast cells and neutrophils that initiate the inflammatory response while NK (natural killer cells) are activated in response to macrophage-derived cytokines that secrete IFN (interferon) and TNF (tumor necrotic factor).

Acting as floating sentinels in our blood and lymph, WBCs unleash chemicals and phagocytes as they fight a viral infection, often according to a cytokine's nudge.

A cytokine, like interferon, is a signaling molecule or chemical messenger that binds to the surface of a cell to get it to do their bidding.

Toll-like receptors (TLRs) act as an alarm system for both the innate and adaptive systems. These are abundant on the surface of macrophages, neutrophils as well as on the epithelial cells lining the lung and gut. TLRs are "pattern recognition proteins" that discriminate between self and non-self. They recognize a wide range of viruses leading to the production of various cytokines including ROS (reactive oxygen species) and AMPs (antimicrobial peptides)[4] all prime members of the antiviral league.

Loitering in almost every corner of the body, the WBCs monitor and defend us from pathogens: they engulf, digest, and spray as well as excrete waste generated. Once they process the pathogen or antigen (*i.e.* virus) they migrate to a draining lymph node, presenting this disassembled virus (if a viral infection) to a T lymphocyte for further removal by the adaptive immune response. (This will then generate antigen-specific cytotoxic T cells that can clear the infection through T1 or the cell-mediated side of the adaptive system.)

Cytokines such as interferon, the key cytokine that mediates antiviral responses, were discovered by Isaacs and Lindenmann in 1957, getting its name from their function to "interfere" in viral replication. Other cytokines include IL-1, IL-6, IL-8 and IL-12, produced at the early stage of the innate side of the immune equation with an emphasis on the enzyme AMP (antimicrobial peptide), also part of our ancient defense system.[4-8]

Among other actions, AMP (aka AMPK) decreases inflammation (remember inflammation is the beginning of any disease process) and normalizes cellular energy that is essential for homeostasis (cell stability). Detoxification or autophagy (remember essential in any healing) plays a role in gut health as well as the production of mitochondria (essential to recovery due to being the main power source of the cell). AMPs inhibit NFkB[6,8] the primary activator of chronic inflammation...well, the "ands" could go on and on leaving us with the understanding and perhaps excitement of a direct link to regulating our immune systems through natural activity.

As we've learned, cytokines play an important, yet conflicting role, in how the body deals with infection, influencing the white blood cells,[6,9] and instructing immune cells what to do in order to knock out the infection.[7] Besides fever, they also trigger inflammation, runny nose, body aches, and having woken up the other cells—neutrophils, macrophages, dendritic, T cells—attack infected cells and ultimately clear the virus from the body.

Cytokines are also responsible for the feeling of chills and/or heat: they migrate to the brain, activating heat-generating areas in order to promote a faster viral clearance. Unfortunately, in 1918 and seemingly now in COVID-19, they can rev up immune activity too well. Too many pro-inflammatory cytokines create a cytokine storm that goes on to damage organs especially the lungs and kidneys, often resulting in death.[9]

If you take nothing else from this book, remember the lesson from the nasty cytokine storms of the Great Flu of 1918 so that we can implement what is at the heart of the deaths of COVID-19: the need for proper nutrition and sufficient detoxification.

THE COMPLEMENT SYSTEM

Another first line of defense is the complement system,[10-12] a complex network that can elicit another highly efficient and normally tightly regulated system against an infectious organism like a virus. It activates enzyme reactions through proteins and glycoproteins synthesized by liver cells, blood monocytes, tissue macrophages and the epithelial cells in the genitourinary and gastrointestinal tracts. This system gets rid of viruses by lysing them, activating inflammation, coating particles and clearing debris, as well as tagging them through opsonization that increases the chance of viruses being gobbled up.

Research is turning to the C3 and C5 complements of the complement system to find how these can be inhibited. Many plants are showing promise. These are just a few: licorice (*Glycyrrhiza glabra*); *Juglans* spp. that has high amounts of flavonoids including quercetin; propolis from bees; the popular Ayurvedic toothpaste neem (*Azadirachta indica,*) Morinda (a hit in Congo for arthritis); rosemary, aloe, and so many more.[10] Are you seeing how we can influence our immune system?

THE LYMPHATIC SYSTEM

Another player in the initial vigil is the lymphatic system that runs alongside our arteries and veins, drawing waste, bacteria, decaying blood cells and water into it. Lymph nodes are tiny immune stations that are tightly packed with our heroes, the white blood cells.

Lymphatic vessels surround all of our organs, creating an intricate network of garbage collectors that stream toward the cisterna chyli that lies on the right side of the spine near the stomach. Waste and water collect here before being propelled by the diaphragm to the left thoracic duct that empties into the left subclavian vein (the right thoracic duct drains the head and neck into the right subclavian vein) and then into the heart. Yada yada yada...but it's cool right? (It's also important to know that two thirds of lymph is produced in the liver and intestines, organs we can further help through nutrients, lifestyle and detoxification.)

The flow through this lymphatic vasculature moves forward only when it is pressed as in massage, when we move and with enzymes from fresh fruit and vegetables. (All things we can have a say in!) Otherwise it is even more slow and passive, and not affected by the heart that takes direction only from the movement of our diaphragm, our breathing. Contrarily, even at death, the lymph system will continue to pull in fluids for up to twenty-four hours.

The thymus and the spleen are two major organs that belong to the lymphatic system. Although the thymus, large at childhood, shrinks after puberty, it leaves an imprint on the immune system. It is where lymphocytes mature and receive their immunological instruction before being released into the bloodstream. The spleen, on the other hand, receives and cleanses both lymph and blood 'til death do we part (although it is true a person does not have to have a spleen but by knowing what it does we can act accordingly and keep our bodies as clean as possible.)

As blood flows into the spleen, worn out red blood cells and platelets are removed. The spleen transports and transforms food and fluid from the digestive tract to the tissues.

Except for a sluggish tired feeling that we may not know is coming from a drainage problem in the lymph system, a sewage backup so to speak, one symptom we do feel is a swollen lymph node. This stagnation can be very harmful as waste is not being removed and the blood vessels that parallel the lymph can become toxic, depriving us of optimal perfusion of oxygen.

Remember, optimum lymphatic function is essential to healing. To be healthy the lymph must be freely moving, easily and effectively drawing waste from the tissues, blood, and interstitial fluids. With too much fat or junk food or environmental toxins this system can easily get clogged like the liver. Bioflavonoids in raw fruits and vegetables with deep color can heal damaged lymph vessels. Naturally occurring enzymes, and antioxidants like Vitamins A, C, E and minerals such as selenium and manganese, in vegetables and fruit help lymph flow.

The GI, liver and lungs round out our award ceremony with GI symptoms such as diarrhea, vomiting, and abdominal pain common manifestations in a viral infection and can be a hallmark of a severe infection.[12]

Named for their "tree like" or dendritic shapes, the dendritic cells play a crucial role in both destroying the virus and carrying it to nearby lymph nodes, activating the T lymphs on the adaptive side of the immune response.

THE ADAPTIVE SYSTEM

Made up of lymphocytes—T cells and B cells—the adaptive or acquired system is concerned with clearing the infection. While slower in development in its initial meeting with a pathogen like a virus and can take a week to respond, it is highly specific and effective at destroying the virus again in the future due to making antibodies.

This system includes: 1) the Th1 cell-mediated response that assures the attachment to the antigen—the invading virus for our purpose—by destroying or tagging it for destruction by other cells and eliminating it through detox pathways; and 2) the Th2 humoral response that produces antibodies that we won't be concerned with until after the infection. This is what a vaccine stimulates but without Th1, meaning there is no elimination stage so all the toxic particles that should be sent to the lymph system are not.

Two of the most important T lymphocytes are helper Ts, also called CD4, and killer Ts, CD8. The job of killer Ts is to search out body cells that are infected with viruses and go in for the kill. Helper T cells are said to be the glue of the immune system because their secretions rally the troops—the phagocytic cells, B lymphs and Killer Ts. Another subset, T regs (T regulatory cells), help control the T helper and killer cells by stopping them from over-reacting and attacking the body itself thus causing autoimmunity.

An important job for the lymphocytes is to calm the immune system once the white blood cells win the battle against the marauding virus returning the immune system to a "quiet vigil." Memory cells from B lymph are left to identify any pathogens, making sure to enlist antibodies. These are the cells that confer long lasting immunity. (About ten trillion B cells stream through the blood and lymph, one fifth of all the proteins found in blood, but viruses are too protected once inside cells for B cells to get to them.)

It's the cell-mediated response of the adaptive system that is the sickness, having been informed by what is termed the inflammasome.

THE INFLAMMASOME

Once a virus enters the body the signaling platform of the inflammasome arises in response to cell disruption such as irregular ion influxes (*i.e.* sodium and potassium balance) and/or mitochondria dysfunction. This process leads to activation of protease enzymes and pro-inflammatory cytokines that will interfere with protein secretions and initiate cell death as we have seen in the function of white blood cells.

In influenza or COVID-19, this period is normally marked by a fever, the body's attempt to kill the virus, mucus that is sneezed or blown out the nose and coughing.[12,13]

The inflammasome marks the beginning of being sick. Note: if our immune system is really diminished, not working properly, we may not get sick at all because our body is not able to mount a defense, *i.e.* that's how depleted the body is, you may very well be on the path to death. This is why it's important to maintain adequate levels of nutrients especially Vitamin D,[14] sweat through hot drinks, use hydrotherapy of various kinds including sauna, and take herbs and/or homeopathy to promote the healing pathway of expectoration of mucus and dead cells. Detoxification is mandatory for optimal healing and subsequent wellness and is really what the body through an acute sickness is attempting to do.

With all this knowledge let's whistle some appreciation of what nature does for us.

Clearly, we do not need to panic.

SUMMARY OF OUR NATURAL IMMUNE SYSTEM'S DEFENSE AGAINST AN ATTACKING VIRUS - GIVING YOU EVEN MORE CONFIDENCE IN WHAT YOUR BODY CAN DO:

1. Activation of lung monocytes that become macrophages: these cells swallow (phagocytose) the viruses themselves or the infected cells.
2. Once the viruses and cells are inside the macrophages and dendritic cells, they are broken down into small pieces. These pieces (epitopes) are transported out to the surface of the cells on the outside and allow the killer T cells to inspect and memorize it so they can kill the next infected cell.
3. Other T-cells, called helper, help B-cells to make antibodies against the viruses or the infected cells; thus, effectively tag them for destruction or preventing them from spreading.
4. At the same time T and B memory cells are produced to function as a cellular response to the same or similar infection in the future. That is the reason the next infection can be cleared much faster.
5. At the same time T-regulatory cells are activated as they try to stop over stimulation of the ramped up immune system.[15]
6. The stimulation of the response is dependent on many nutrients such as Vitamin A, D, C, essential fatty acids, trace minerals,[16] as

these factors stimulate the immune system to get rid of the virus; they also make sure that the response does not get out of hand causing excessive damage and sometimes death as in the cytokine storm scenario. The same nutrients stimulate the T regulatory cells to stop the over-stimulation of the immune system[15] while pollution, gluten and high fat diet stop the cells from working properly.[16] Lack of these factors and increase in pollution cause a higher risk of developing chronic infection,[17] inflammation and auto-immune diseases.[18]

UNANSWERED QUESTION

The question remains as to how the virus actually kills the patient; why seasonal influenza kills young and old most of the time yet healthy young adults during the Great Flu of 1918. Was the cause a cytokine storm? It seems the answer may lie in nutrition, pollution, and stress.

And as per COVID-19 one theory of activation of lung disease like ARDS (acute respiratory distress system)[18-20] is the immune cells, activated via PPRs (pattern-recognition receptors) drives the release of pro-inflammatory cytokines and increases permeability at vascular endothelial junctions. These leak, damaging the bronchi, and disrupting the air-blood barrier thus air flow. The damage is due to TMAs, *i.e.* thrombotic microangiopathy, the formation of microscopic blood clots in capillaries and small arteries that presents as hemolytic anemia (destruction of red blood cells), low platelets, and organ damage.

For now, let us look more closely at the possible mechanism of the cytokine storm that killed so many in 1918 and is doing the same during COVID-19.

A severe infection can produce hemorrhage and blood clots in the lungs and be lethal (including to the kidneys) by the following action:

1. When a virus infects the cells of the nose, throat or lungs, the cells send a signal that the protective barrier is breached and there is a need for repair.
2. The blood vessels become leakier, allowing immune cells to pass through to try to stop the damage.
3. A complicated coagulation cascade occurs that culminates with

the activation of fibrin (a protein that plugs up the damage) with the help of thrombin (another protein in the cascade that helps with the coagulation). Platelets or thrombocytes (cells that selflessly give up themselves to plug up the damage) rush to the site of injury and entangle themselves with fibrin to help to contain the damage and release signaling molecules to attract all of the other white blood cells and make the blood vessels even more leakier.

4. At the same time plasmin (a protein in the anti-coagulation pathway) degrades fibrin in order not to create a clot that can block a blood vessel.
5. This dance occurs all over the blood vessels in the lungs or anywhere else where damage is already present. Viral proteins help increase the thrombus formation by stimulating the plasmin protein. (This might be one of the reasons there is a higher risk of heart attack and stroke with the infection and especially after years of being exposed to pollution.)
6. Since the immune system is preoccupied with the clearance of the virus and thrombi, bacterial infection can begin from the resident bacteria that lives in the lung that also promotes the coagulation. If a person is a smoker or exposed to air pollution, the damage from the toxins in the smoke and the air pollution increase the severity of the coagulation and increases the susceptibility to the infection. Probiotics and all of the nutrients we will discuss soon work to repair the damage and stop the immune overstimulation by supporting the blood vessels and the barrier cells in the respiratory tract.

ASSIGNMENT #3

1. Why is the lymph system important?
2. What are the two parts of the immune system?
3. What is a cytokine storm and why is it dangerous?
4. Can you name three activities the white blood cells do to resist a virus?

CHAPTER 4: THE BASICS OF IMMUNE RESISTANCE

Clearly our body's natural immunity is a force to be reckoned with and ancient healing principles coupled with modern applications help focus this innate healing power.

But what are these principles and applications that build resistance and resilience to prevent a viral cascade that may lead to severe illness and even death?

As was discussed in the last chapter there are many factors involved in the deadliest consequence of a viral infection: a cytokine storm. To avoid this from occurring we retain the information of people who have come before us, we learn from past mistakes while remembering that from time infinitum we have lived in a world of microorganisms and in fact have an ancient defense system within us.

We have a pathway and process called autophagy that breaks down and clears debris as the body fights the virus. This relies in large part on a healthy microbiome, the good bacteria that continues to get great press for all it does for our gut, our brain and yes, fighting off a viral infection.

Here are the main processes or substances that are key to surviving a viral infection like influenza or in COVID-19, SARS-CoV-2.

OUR INNER ECOSYSTEM

The majority of bacteria, fungi and viruses are our natural partners that coexist and keep us healthy (remember most viruses are harmless.) These organisms act as a first line of defense so that our bodies interact optimally with the outer world whether this be epithelial surfaces or what is basically a tube, but to the outside, our gastrointestinal tract.

Ensuring a healthy flora in our gut means our microorganisms are happy and in balance. Otherwise our immune response has to work doubly hard as it attempts to right this problem before going on to tackle the virus.

When the body's ecosystem is dysfunctional, harmful bacteria may "overgrow." Coupled with the mucosa infected by the influenza virus, these two factors further promote invasion of pathogenic bacteria, promoting susceptibility to the disease. This is why ingestion of fiber, fermented foods and/or probiotics is essential to maximize immune function, decreasing the chance to become sick with the flu or another viral infection.

If treated with antibiotics when we are children[1] (the reality of most in the Western World) we may be more susceptible to disease as our microbiome and immune system have been altered. And vice versa: a pathogenic virus can set up the lungs to harbor bad bacteria that triggers immune system products like cytokines that produce more damage and destruction.

Basically, the consequence of our guts being out of whack is that our immune system can be so strong it can be harmful. We only want one fire (against the virus) to deal with. Otherwise the immune cells fighting the infection may be more damaging than the virus itself due to the system going into overdrive.

Since eighty percent of our immune system lives in our gut it is essential, we pay attention to what lives there and what keeps us healthy.

A WORD ON PROBIOTICS (MORE IN FOOD SECTION)

The theory of autointoxication is attributed to the Russian scientist and discoverer of "probiotics in yogurt," M. Elie Metchnikoff in the early 20th century, who worked at the Pasteur Institute in Paris. He believed putrefactive microbes produced toxic compounds in the gut, substances like phenols and indoles, which are reabsorbed by the intestinal walls, initiating the disease process. He hypothesized that we could normalize bowel health and prolong life by replacing toxic bacteria with lactic acid bacteria, using sour milk, as well as adding lactic bacilli to vegetable and animal broths.

Any probiotic worth its salt helps maintain intestinal microbial health, enhances digestion of food, promotes B vitamin synthesis and supports the immune system. It decreases gas and bloating which can be a lifesaver in terms of health and vanity.

As newborns we get dosed with beneficial bacteria going through the birth canal, flora necessary for gut health,[5] hence our immune system. Unfortunately, life interferes, and many things disrupt this healthy colonization of bacteria. From heavy metals, chlorinated water, junk food, unfettered emotion, so much throws off the balance.

Research is showing they detoxify heavy metals.[2-4]

This is great news as we are contaminated daily through food, water, and air by a range of chemicals and heavy metals such as lead, cadmium, arsenic, chromium, and mercury and are in vaccines as adjuvants. These interfere with metabolic processes and cause disease.

Lactobacillus and *Bifidobacterium* species,[5,6] living in the mouth, gut and vagina, can bind the environmental toxins, lead and cadmium, hold onto them 'til we poop them out. *L. rhamnosus* reduces the bioaccumulation of mercury and arsenic. And *lactobacillus* can transform chromium to its less toxic form.

VITAMINS C and D

For optimal health generally we need to keep a balance of vitamins and minerals. Vitamins C and D particularly are so important to beat back a virus, and increasing them before, during or after, causes no harm.

According to research, there has not been a single virus that has not been inactivated by a large dose of Vitamin C according to many including Frederick Klenner, M.D., called the father of the clinical applications of Vitamin C.[7]

Vitamin C's bioavailability is very high, meaning because of its simple chemical structure, it can get into all nooks and crannies of the body. Wiggling into both intracellular and extracellular spaces, it directly contacts the virus and through other helpers basically blows it to smithereens, disabling viral replication. The ability to get inside the cell is called the "Fenton reaction." Vitamin C also stimulates the antiviral cytokine, interferon, and antibody production.

My favorite form is liposomal Vitamin C. (Liposomal means fat soluble, this enables it to get into cells even easier and so detox faster.)

Vitamin D deficiency is linked to respiratory infections such as TB, bronchiolitis, and pneumonia, the leading cause of death in children around the world and the major concern in any viral infection. It is shown to be prophylactic for Influenza A virus, according to Gerry Schwalfenberg, M.D. in Canadian Family Physician.[8] He is critical of the antivirals NIs, neuraminidases as he's seen it cause the following symptoms in the elderly nursing home: vomiting, diarrhea, confusion, hallucinations, delirium and a decline in cognition. Alternatively, he sees dramatic resolves of flu within 48 hours by giving a high dose of Vitamin D, up to 50, 000 IU or 10,000 TID for two to three days.

We have the research to show Vitamin D helps calm a cytokine storm.[8,9] Other studies show it is beneficial against colds and influenza - both A and B - and in time, we will know definitively about SARS-CoV-2.

STRESS

When stress goes beyond what is necessary it affects the adrenal cortex.[10] This impedes the body's ability to store blood sugar (glycogen) in the liver properly and so our blood sugar drops during the night. When this happens, the brain signals the adrenal glands to release adrenaline and cortisol into the bloodstream. These hormones direct fat cells to the liver so the fat can be turned into sugar.

As Michael Gerber MD, HMD, wrote in *Townsend Letter for Doctors*, October 2014: "The body doesn't die from want of sugar, but there is adrenaline release. It is like trying to sleep on speed, awakening the individual whose mind then goes to the unresolved problems of the day and aggravates the stress response."

There are various substances to suppress this including licorice, Vitamin C and B but the best thing to do is increasing parasympathetic activity (meditation, gentle yoga, singing), exercising and getting into the sun or taking Vitamin D during the day.

SEX AND IGA

We rarely speak of the benefits of sex—orgasms and loving touch—but they can induce higher levels of Immunoglobulin A,[11] our body's first line of defense that acts on mucous membranes. IgAs fight off invading microorganisms at their entry point, whether nose, skin or other portal, leading to reduced need, even to zero, for the rest of your immune system to get involved.

And if you are never in the mood, think of eliminating grains and sugars of all kinds as high levels of blood sugar can turn off sex hormones.

SLEEP

Sleep may be the most important determining factor in regaining and maintaining health. Proper amount of restful sleep makes sure that our immune system functions properly without being over or under reactive.[10] The pineal gland supplies the brain with sulfur, a necessary detoxification substance, while sleeping at night, as we shall see. And adding melatonin for more than circadian rhythm helps fend off the virus.

If you have tried almost everything in all the books and blogs about better sleep think about trying blue light glasses that contain pigments that absorb wavelengths emitted by artificial lights and screens. This will allow for more production of natural melatonin. Thirty minutes outside after waking up in the morning, enjoying your day (increasing serotonin) will also augment melatonin.

GET MOVING/ EXERCISE

Exercise makes it easier to sleep. It increases oxygen and other nutrients to tissue as well as moves the lymphatic system, the body's garbage disposal. However, be careful not to over exercise, especially if there is an epidemic on the horizon. Over-exercising taxes the adrenals and the immune system causing a higher suitability to infections.[12]

HYDRATION

You know what happens when a plant doesn't get water, but what happens if we don't drink enough water? Just about the same...we start to wilt. We may not realize that's why a headache came on or our backs started to hurt and so on, but we need water to hydrate every single cell in our body. Normal everyday functions use water and we lose it through urination, perspiration, and bowel movements. It's so easy to not get enough water when we are hot or have a fever and that's when we need to double up our efforts to keep hydrated. This is even more necessary when diarrhea and vomiting is involved. The lungs can't function properly without being thoroughly hydrated. Did you know that every time you exhale you lose water? When sick, not being hydrated properly causes an increase in mucous concentration in the nose, throat and the lungs, which in turn increases an inability to clear the infection.

During any acute febrile (*i.e.* marked by a fever) disease it is essential that mucous membranes and the skin remain moist. Mucous is filled with IgA-type antibodies and this increases immunity.

Electrolytes keep us balanced. These are minerals in our body that have an electric charge like sodium, potassium, magnesium, calcium, phosphate, and chloride. All cells need them. And especially because much of our modern soil is depleted, we need to make sure we add minerals to our diets even when well. You can get them from the foods you eat and fluids you drink.

The fact is, you don't need sports drinks to do this with their high level of sugar or artificial sugar, artificial flavors and colors. Alkaline water is more beneficial as it hydrates faster – simply add a wedge of lemon or lime, perhaps a sprinkle of sea or Himalayan salt to filtered water.

Hydration may be the deal breaker in getting better quickly or not. It's allowing fluid to wash out your cells so to speak. Ensuring water is continuously available and sipped on, especially for the elderly is an absolute. To begin, teas are fine as long as they are not too stimulating. There is a misconception that teas are benign and can be drunk as much as a person desires: however, teas contain biochemicals that have anti-bacterial, fungal, and viral effects. When consumed in excess they may cause dysfunction of the microbiome, predisposing the person to infections. Moderation is important.

HYGIENE HYPOTHESIS

Another important factor that helps support a healthy immune system is the hygiene hypothesis.[13-15] This states that excessive cleanliness we find in the 21st Century interrupts the normal development of the immune system and that this is a reason allergies are through the roof these days. Modern advances like sanitation and the eradication of parasitic infections can be detrimental to our immune system, as may be the delayed introduction of more common allergenic foods.

Westernized countries with small families in urban areas are most at risk. The microflora we need has been swept away by a thousand cleansers. We no longer get our hands dirty. Of course, developing countries have other problems, like sewage or polyculture (especially in Asia) that can breed disease. We need a happy balance of good bugs to be healthy, ensuring the delicate balance in our gut where our digestion begins.[14, 15]

So, what about today in the COVID-19 era? What can we do to help people stay well? How do we prevent suffering and death? Does the cytokine storm have roots in poor nutrition and a toxic environment that is contributing to blood clots and oxygen deprivation?

You can bet on it.

The next section turns to historical facts that impeded optimal health delivery and what we must learn from it, particularly in 2020, to ensure optimal health to move forward with confidence to fight this emerging coronavirus, SARS-CoV-2 or a possible super influenza virus.

ASSIGNMENT #4

1. What is the hygiene hypothesis?
2. Discuss the word microbiome and how it applies to your gut.
3. What is and how does autophagy contribute to healing a viral infection?
4. Name five free activities you can implement to boost your immune system.

PART TWO: WHAT HAPPENED?

CHAPTER 5: A PARADIGM SHIFT

Fifty years ago, the physicist, not a philosopher by trade, Thomas Kuhn, introduced the phrase "paradigm shift" through his book, *The Structure of Scientific Revolutions*, one of the most cited academic books of all time. Without getting too detailed, his theory addressed the obstacles to how science advances, or doesn't. He argued that science does not move steadily on (aka progress) with growing evidence adding to the accumulation of research to offer us the best of what we know of the natural world including our own bodies. Instead "he saw discontinuities—a set of alternating 'normal' and 'revolutionary' phases in which communities of specialists in particular fields are plunged into periods of turmoil, uncertainty and angst."[1]

This is not unlike what we have gone through in the last one hundred years, as the general public has been both blessed and cursed by modern medicine. With influences initially generated by the elites at the financial helm—the robber barons—the dominant system of medicine they backed, in all its obvious benefits, has also given us the quick-fix pill-popping mentality that has led to antibiotic resistance, an opioid epidemic, vaccine injury and other catastrophes.

There are many theoretical constructs to explain health and disease and none more evident than the last three hundred years in America. We need simply turn to Hippocrates or Galen or Hahnemann or even Samuel Thomson or Juliette Bairacli Levy to get a glimpse of different "filters," different ideas and methods intended to balance the body and mind. From bloodletting, purging, so-called "heroic" medicine, to the infinitesimal doses of homeopathy or the applications of plants, there have been many theories, many competing methodologies throughout the continent.

It was, in fact, the constraints of medical education that ultimately changed everything.

ROOTS OF EXCLUSION

With little formal training, North American doctors in the nineteenth century were mocked by their European counterparts for not having medical schools; instead, doctors trained through apprenticeships. It was not a time of respect or prosperity for physicians and this disturbed them. Medical societies or associations formed, each hoping to advance their particular system of medicine. The doctors who used bloodletting, calomel and other so-called "heroic" measures in their practice called themselves "regulars." Then there were those given the name "irregulars"—this included medical and Eclectic doctors who employed homeopathy or botanical medicine (herbs); herbalists, midwives and other forms of medical practice were pushed off the menu. Yet three-quarters of medical doctors successfully practiced homeopathy as their mainstay of practice. (The yellow fever epidemics in New Orleans at that time are an example. Records were kept and the homeopaths had a much higher success rate than the allopaths as the "regulars" were also called.)

Many physicians, during this time, chose to complete their medical studies abroad in schools in Great Britain, France and notably, Germany, a country whose influence of scientific discovery led to a lopsided approach to wellness as we will see.

The "regulars" or allopaths, threatened by the "irregulars" particularly midwives who impinged upon their obstetrics practice, wanted exclusivity in order to make a higher wage. They discouraged anyone other than a "heroic practitioner," creating a climate where others who were in line with nature (remember *Vis Medicatrix Naturae,* the healing power of nature), were called "alternative" practitioners, a situation that continues to this day, as anyone other than allopaths are called "alternative" practitioners.

It is hard to fathom that this division only commenced from greed, but this was the motive according to several historians including E. Richard Brown, who wrote an entire book about it in his 1972 book, *Rockefeller Medicine Men.*

Brown shows that the relationship entwining science, education and industrialization began mid nineteenth century when the newly minted industrialists and presidents of medical schools aligned their interests. The first national scientific congress was held in 1844 and the audience was told that the little science America was investigating didn't have the support it needed by institutions of the day and had few professional scientists.

Already shamed by Europe's disdain for North America's lack of medical schools, these attendees clamored for backing from philanthropists who would see that a certain type of personnel was needed for the growing industrial and corporate economy that they hoped would now include medical schools reflecting their vision.

The backdrop at this time included the end of the American Civil War. "The Civil War not only freed the black slaves from the legal bonds of slavery. It also freed the hand of the Northern capital to extend throughout the nation the industrial transformation it had begun mainly north of the Ohio River. As the 'underground railroad' was the vehicle and symbol of freedom for ante-bellum slaves, the iron railroad was the vehicle and symbol of industrialization and the ascending capitalist class…As the railroads were used increasingly to move troops and supplies for the Union armies, they helped extend and integrate the marketplace…coordinated across the continent."[2]

This fed the continued rise of the wealthy railroad, oil and steel men—including Andrew Carnegie and JD Rockefeller, Sr.—who had made their fortunes by supplying the Union armies and would continue to reap exorbitant gains afterwards feeding the needs of a growing nation. And although positive for the economy in general—farm products to emerging markets and raw material like cotton, iron ore and oil to mills or refineries, and steel for new construction of 62,000 miles of new track in the 1860s and 70s—it enabled the men who owned these new corporations to not just make money but to take firm control of the new economy. And that meant, as today, industrial workers were paid as little as possible while craftspeople fell by the wayside as machines took over.

During the time between the Civil War and World War these people who had thrived on individual and community pride, who had owned farms, or created art or crafts, were then drawn into factories. Becoming cogs in a system—even with organized labor—they were exploited and lost to corporations in which the bottom line was not their healthcare or safety but the profit line of the owners. These farmers and townspeople increasingly felt their lives controlled by the financiers in a distant corporate office who gave them little voice.

From 1870 to 1898 the US population grew quickly, and the economy doubled. With enormous political corruption and inside corporations, few laws regulated business. By 1914 what had once been "a playground for European empires" was now the largest industrial nation in the world. People lived grand lives at the expense of those in tremendous poverty. The pro-business Congress and courts seemed to overlook this until labor unions forced its hand.

J. D. Rockefeller, the richest Baptist in the world, was in terrible health by his fifties in 1889, suffering nervous fatigue, stomach problems, even losing all body hair. He hired the Reverend Frederick T. Gates to run his philanthropy: by then the Rockefeller Foundation included many medical and public health programs.

Eventually, Andrew Carnegie would have a revelation: "The man who dies thus rich dies disgraced," and gave much of his wealth away, but in the meantime, he forced medicine in a limited direction. (William Jewett Tucker, a liberal theologian and later president of Dartmouth College, nailed it in his objection: "I can conceive of no greater mistake, than that of trying to make charity do the work of justice."[3]) Gates, raised in poverty, became disillusioned as a minister, before finding his calling as a businessman, and although he had similar fears to Carnegie, it was Gates' notions and tactics that led Rockefeller's money to focus on transforming social institutions through charity in a capitalist society that in fact was based on self-interest. And we are paying for this today as witnessed in a lopsided healthcare system with roots in corporate capitalism.

Throughout the 1800s, as scientific development increased, calls to reform medical education resounded throughout North America but it was not until 1910 when the Carnegie Foundation commissioned Abraham Flexner (brother Simon was a medical doctor) to survey medical education that the biomedical model became pivotal in its attack on other systems of medicine.

Abraham Flexner—a schoolteacher and educational theorist from Louisville, Kentucky—with N.P. Colwell, the secretary of the AMA Council on Medical Education visited 55 medical schools throughout Canada and the US and Canada, holding the maxim "research was the air we breathed." He had a "ruthless, unforgiving judgment"[2] in advancing medical education.

Gates, who had earlier toured European medical schools and, influenced by William Welch of Johns Hopkins University, became fond of the German model. He was taken with the "hyper-rational system of German science" that would leave out the art in the art and science of medicine. In this way his gold standard mandated laboratories with cadavers and research facilities as a requirement for medical schools but included little else in terms of patient care and the results of this care, turning a blind eye to the natural and humane practices of medicine.

To receive a top grade from Gates and Flexner, the school had to be affiliated with a university and teaching hospital, or you lost funding. This criterion changed medicine drastically. Forty-six medical schools closed between 1910 and 1920 due to an inability to afford research facilities. These schools included homeopathic medical schools (where the research criteria is much different than allopathic, no matter how valid both are) and bankrupted medical training for women and Blacks although the reality also included Jews, Catholics, Italians, the poor, and people who believed the healing power of nature—homeopathy, naturopathic medicine, First Nation/Native American medicine.

As Adrienne Morgan, PhD, in her doctoral thesis[4] states of the American medical school admissions at the time of the Flexner Report, "... the ideal medical student should be white, male and Protestant."

Apparently, the Carnegie Foundation in 1918 wrote the AMA Council on Education that they realized "a grave injustice to black medicine had been done,"[5] but the damage was a fait accompli. (Only two Black schools, Meharry Medical College and Howard University College of Medicine remained untouched.) The attitude to Blacks in medicine thus remained the same since 1872.[3]

Flexner's book length report, *Medical Education in the United States and Canada* (aka *The Flexner Report)* has affected our lives in ways we cannot imagine. The present opioid epidemic is a case in point. As well as in COVID-19.

This transformation of medicine left most people ignoring natural principals while ensuring the patents and profits of lab created products. It excluded from its final analysis both a measure of clinical caring and the body's inherent ability to heal. And it would be at the root of the deadly cytokine storms of the Great Flu of 1918.

As an honest Kentucky politician, Joseph C.S. Blackburn, one of the fiercest critics of US Imperialism in the late 1800s, added to the aphorism attributed to Percy Bysshe Shelley, "The rich grow richer, the poor become poorer" with "and the nation trembles."[2]

Just as today, and we can include the color of our skin, our gender and our sexual orientation, all liabilities in a white man's world to the growing discord in conventional or allopathic medicine.

RELATION TO COVID-19

During the Industrial Age, leading up to the Great Flu, people were forced off their land to live in crowded cities without proper sanitation and without the bounty of vegetables and fruits and clean water. The Land Enclosure Acts in England is an excellent example of the loss of benefit of not living on the land as the agricultural practice became one of raising pigs and chickens in close quarters and in proximity to other humans. This created the perfect environment for quickened mutation and transmission of viruses, including influenza, that are able to infect humans and cause disease.

The crowding of soldiers in trenches and barracks is likened to this and is one theory why the cytokine storm occurred in the 1918 pandemic, killing predominantly young and healthy soldiers, and adversely affecting pregnant women. It seems then and today, poor nutrition with a diminished availability of vegetables and fruits plays a huge part in keeping an immune system balanced with the stress of being in the army depleting already low vitamin C and D as well as other essential nutrients,[6-10] thus making them more susceptible to the infection of a newly mutated virus. (See Table 1 in the Appendix B for complete details on a sample soldier's diet at the time.)

Women's nutritional status suffers during pregnancy, and especially on a poor diet at that time during urbanization.[6-10] Children were not breastfed as much as in the past and those who were most likely did not receive an optimal amount of nutrients to develop properly which could change how their genes could operate after birth. Artificial baby formulas with poor nutrient content were introduced and are notorious for being detrimental to the gut microbiome and the immune system.

Other factors included heavy coal burning and other sources of heavy pollution.[11]

These pollutants suppress and/or dysregulate the immune system and irritate the mucosal lining promoting infections as well as damaging the gut microbiome.

And we can't forget that a plethora of viruses and bacteria caused significant morbidity and mortality rates at this time: "typhoid fever, typhus fever, relapsing fever, malaria, smallpox, measles, scarlet fever, pertussis, diphtheria, croup, influenza, military fever, Asiatic cholera, cholera nostras, dysentery, plague, yellow fever, leprosy, erysipelas, purulent infection, septicemia, glanders, anthrax, rabies, tetanus, mycoses, tuberculosis, rickets, syphilis, gonococcal infection, other 'epidemic, endemic, or infectious diseases,' acute articular rheumatism (1900 through 1920)."[12]

Current science underscores that for such gruesome deaths in the pandemic of 1918 to occur a combination of factors led to the higher death rates including the terror of an immune system phenomenon, a cytokine storm, that causes severe blood coagulation. (See Chapter 4) As we learned, cytokines are immune-regulatory proteins that in their attempt to kill the virus can endanger the host, acting up to one thousand times normal activity that can lead to death of the host (that would be us.) Remember, this overreaction can be pacified by Vitamins C and D and other nutrients readily available in good nutrition.

IMPOSED BIGOTRY

To say that the Flexner Report and its roots have affected our health as a nation over the last one hundred and twenty years is a grave understatement. Abraham Flexner's arrogance in determining that all systems of medicine must have research facilities as he imagined was not a paradigm shift but imposed bigotry. Funded by oil and steel barons, Flexner decided the fates of medical schools based on an incomplete theory of assuming medicine or healing needed only be aligned with facilities that emphasized laboratory research. It was also at this time that patent medicine became fixed—a formula could be owned—from which the pharmaceutical companies base their profits.

The Rockefeller and Carnegie Foundations, knowingly or not, honestly or dishonestly, placed a stranglehold on the practice of medicine in this country, casting natural medicine to the wind. They have pushed and cajoled and strong-armed medical professionals and the public away from natural healing to become dependent on pills or surgical intervention. I once had a patient ask, "But how do I heal without a pill?"

Science is absolutely wonderful, but it can be manipulated in medicine as we see in the reality of opioid abuse today due to the fact we have not learned a complete approach to healthcare. Today, more than ever, we need to understand the root of the exclusion of other "filters," those system of medicines that are not alternatives but must stand as answers—along with political, social and environmental solutions—that can help us dialogue and detoxify historical realities (poverty, racism, sexism and cytokine storms) that led to a disregard of what our bodies and minds are capable through natural means. One cannot overemphasize the past and current efforts of the oil and steel industries to profligate a practice of medicine that draws on resources to promote its own selfish endeavors. (A conflict of interest indeed.)

Because not only were the robber barons who funded the Flexner's Report responsible for bypassing valid and necessary systems of medicine, they were guilty of owning factories, mills and mines that led to pollution, contamination, unsafe working conditions and untold deaths.

Despite their best efforts to withstand change, workplace regulations were finally created. In 1907 the Tillman Act had Congress banning corporations from funding federal companies and in 1947 the Taft-Hartley Act extended the ban to labor unions. But these laws were hard to enforce and so the wealthy continued to influence the country's politics. (As they continue to do with political lobbyists like Citizens United.)

In terms of medicine, the Flexner Report assumed medical systems such as homeopathic (practiced by medical doctors and not without its prejudices), naturopathic, chiropractic, midwifery, botanical (indigenous, Samuel Thompson, Eclectic medical doctors), and traditional Chinese medicine (TCM) were inferior. They are not alternatives but part of a continuum of care that every person has a right to receive.

NATUROPATHIC MEDICINE

The naturopathic practice of medicine may go back little more than a century, but its roots run thousands of years as it embraces almost every culture that developed a healing system. It's a bit of a tangled web why naturopathic medicine became a distinct profession with schools and licensed doctors while homeopathy faded away, out of conventional medical schools but Flexner's Report did put an end to homeopathic medical schools that, losing its legal footing with allopathy, never recovered to a licensable degree. Thankfully, Naturopathic Medicine, based on the vitalism of both Nature Cure and Homeopathy, kept this extraordinary yet highly disparaged energetic system alive in America including homeopathic pharmacies like Boerke and Tafel and Boiron.

It was Dr. Benedict Lust who brought Kneipp hydrotherapy from Germany to America and founded the first school of naturopathy, as he named it, with his wife Louisa Stroebel Lust. Its first graduating class of 1902 had a curriculum that included botanical medicine, homeopathy, manipulation, hydrotherapy, physiotherapy, nutrition and psychology, mind-body medicine. A distinct primary health care profession, it includes modern and traditional, scientific and empirical methods. It emphasizes prevention and optimal health through therapeutic methods and substances that recognize the inherent self-healing process that is ordered and intelligent and depends on harmony with nature.

Naturopathic physicians treat the cause (*tolle causam*), removing the underlying causes of illness rather than merely eliminate or suppress symptoms. The saying First do no harm (*primum non nocere*) is what we all swear to go by while avoiding the risk of harmful side effects. Another one of our absolutes is to treat the whole person, taking into account the physical, emotional, mental as well as the patient's community and environment.

The word doctor comes from the word teacher (*docere*). We educate patients on their specific condition or disease, encouraging an active role in their health care, to work with the doctor rather than be told what to do with no understanding of treatment.

At one time, like homeopathic medical schools, naturopathic medical colleges were numerous. NDs were licensed in most states until the 1940s when the rise of pharmaceutical drugs and medical technology offered people what they felt was a superior treatment. Almost all schools offering an ND degree closed their doors until 1956 when the National College of Naturopathic Medicine (now National University of Natural Medicine) was founded in Portland, Oregon. In 1979 three of its graduates founded John Bastyr College of Naturopathic Medicine (now Bastyr University) in Seattle, Washington. (In 2012 Bastyr expanded with a campus in San Diego.)

Our letters are ND for naturopathic doctor or NMD for naturopathic medical doctor in Arizona and California. I am a naturopathic medical doctor, board certified in homeopathy, and trained as a primary care doctor. In most licensable states and provinces, we are called naturopathic physicians. In the state of California and the province of Quebec licenses are granted to traditional naturopaths in a two-tier system, and although not trained as primary care doctors, adhere to the same philosophy.

Despite the uneven nature of the medical field, there are several currently licensable systems of medicine that are holistic and integrative, staying true to nature's hand in healing. These are naturopathic medicine; traditional Chinese medicine including acupuncture; traditional osteopathic medicine, and chiropractic medicine. Unfortunately, homeopathic medicine and botanical medicine are not licensable on their own and are practiced within one of these systems.

It is only in the last decades that there are now standalone homeopathic schools, including the Canadian Academy of Homeopathy founded by a naturopathic physician Dr. André Saine.

ASSIGNMENT #5

1. What does the term "paradigm shift" refer to?
2. What is a robber baron? Name two. How has their influence shaped history?
3. What year and what was the Flexner report? Discuss its effect on medicine and your life in 2020.
4. What does *vis medicatrix naturae* mean?

CHAPTER 6: THE BURDEN OF ENVIRONMENTAL TOXINS

The year 2020 marked approximately 75 years since man-made chemicals began their audacious climb into our every cell. The advertising phrase, Better Health Through Chemistry, from the 1950s turned out to be dead wrong. Perhaps the intent was good but what society failed to take into account was the toxic effect of these chemicals on our body's regulatory processes that depend on healthy enzymes and molecules to do their work safely and efficiently.

In fact, one factor in the Great Flu of 1918 is that the industrial revolution at the turn of the 19th Century and the beginning of the 20th consisted of heavy coal burning and other sources of pollution that can suppress and/or dysregulate the immune system and irritate the mucosal lining, promoting infections as well as in the gut microbiome.[1] Over a century later harmful effects of many man-made chemicals particularly in RoundUp® such as its active ingredient, glyphosate, are disastrous to our health. According to MIT researcher, Stephanie Seneff,[2] this may be one cause of COVID-19 patients becoming so ill. (Note: so-called "inert" ingredients such as POEA in the weed killer may be far more toxic than glyphosate.)

Allopathic medicine, by and large, has opted to ignore the effect of the 80,000 chemicals let loose on our bodies and minds with symptoms overlooked that may be due to a toxin. Whether from food, contaminated soil or water, or the air we breathe, our bodies can become overwhelmed; our general detox system through the liver, gut, kidneys and skin unable to metabolize and excrete toxins completely. Heavy metals and pesticides invade and become a scourge on our thyroid, brains[3] and our innate immune system.[4] Aluminum is added to all vaccines and has been known since 1911 to be harmful. [5-6]

In 2016, H.R. 2576 (House of Representatives), a chemical safety bill introduced by Senator Frank R. Lautenberg, was passed with bipartisan support under Obama's presidency. It was the first government attempt at updating regulations to toxic chemicals since the Toxic Substances Control Act of 1976 (yikes, forty years)!

The EPA is now obligated to test the safety of the 2000 chemicals introduced yearly but at only 20 a year, with a seven year deadline, and with a total of 60,000 out of the total 80,000 synthetic chemicals in need of testing, it's going to be a torturously slow overhaul.

However the incomprehensible Supreme Court's 5 to 4 ruling on January 21, 2010 in response to Citizens United vs. FEC (Federal Election Commission) became law, lifting the restriction on electoral campaign donations. It threw out the corporate and union ban on political financial contributions agreeing that it violated the First Amendment. This has led to the ability on the part of oil and gas companies or any corporation that would gain from exploiting the environment, to generate unlimited ads along with other ways to influence the electorate. (Super PACs are "not so shadow" political parties with access to these unlimited donations.)

This decision pleased present-day robber barons, or rather fossil fuel barons to the core. They could now use their billions of dollars to influence our health through contaminating it, making us ill. Unbelievable! You've heard it before, and you'll keep on hearing it: oil and coal and chemical waste from pulp mills has damaged the environment and our bodies to an unprecedented degree.

Two Texan brothers, Charles and the late David Koch, inheritors of tremendous wealth, are examples of fossil fuel barons, exhibiting modern ruthlessness and greed. Their enormous fortune comes from "extractive" energy that they own without having to answer to public shareholders. Their lobbying against government regulations to lower carbon emissions is putting not only our health but the planet, on notice. And the way they are doing this is, to my sensibility, evil. Apparently, as a child, Charles Koch "when called upon to split a treat with his brothers said with a 'wise guy grin: I just want my fair share—which is all of it."[7] What's most egregious is the extreme pollution resulting from their enterprises with their ability to hide from scrutiny while poisoning us all. [8–11]

Dan Glickman, a Senior Fellow at the Bipartisan Policy Center, said of the Kochs: "Their political theory is nothing more than a rationalization for self-interest." Even Warren Buffett said, "There's class warfare all right. But it's my class, the rich class, that's making war, and we're winning."

One example of Charles' activities is CSE—Citizens for a Sound Economy—a non-profit and therefore tax-exempt group based on neo-conservatism policies, with no real members, and classified, and this is truly heinous, as educational. Charles' contribution of $7.9 million helped CSE kill Bill Clinton's energy tax bill that would have had fossil fuel companies pay while renewable energies would have been exempt. Its spinoff, Citizens for the Environment, resorting to ignorance is bliss, called acid rain and other environmental issues "myths." It has now reinvented itself as FreedomWorks.

Journalist and author Jane Mayer calls these kinds of groups: "...a new kind of weapon in the arsenal of several of America's biggest businesses—a fake populist movement secretly manufactured by corporate sponsors not grassroots. These groups have come to be called Astroturf," a fitting name.

Another example of environmental malfeasance happened in Arkansas. Georgia Pacific Paper, a mill owned by Koch Industries, dumped chemical waste resulting in cancer and birth defects with no penalty and or one easily affordable. Stories like this are endless.

In 2012 the EPAs Toxic Release Inventory database documented the toxic and carcinogenic output of 8000 American companies with Koch Industries being the #1 producer of toxic waste in the United States.[7]

It is the Gilded Age tarnished to the nth degree.

POTENTIAL DAMAGE

Harmful environmental substances cause immense oxidative damage[12-18] through free radicals aka unpaired electrons, poisoning our bodies and the environment through reckless industrial standards that deny this reality. This is why we must ingest high amounts of antioxidants like Vitamin C to stay well as well as eat organic food, use pure cosmetics and laundry products and so on. It is our duty to ourselves, our children and the planet to right this shortsighted wrong and create a daily detox.

For more information, check out groups like the Environmental Working Group (ewg.org).

WHAT THE PROBLEM IS

Toxins can affect us by displacing minerals: the toxin sits on a receptor site that is meant for a mineral or a hormone. Endocrine disruptors are rampant in modern life and any system in the body controlled by hormones can be affected. Most of us are deficient in minerals due to poor or toxic soil and so it becomes a vicious cycle.

Heavy metals such as aluminum or mercury or a pesticide like glyphosate, can cross the blood brain barrier. These become neurotoxins, damaging the brain.[3] Or they can disrupt our gut microbiome, leading to devastating effects from metabolic disruption. These possibilities can be especially destructive to a baby or child whose brain is in development and influenced by the gastrointestinal link (aka gut-brain axis).[4]

Whether an xenoestrogen (a substance that mimics estrogen), heavy metal like lead or mercury, pesticide ike glyphosate, a plasticizer like BPA (bisphenol A) in our soil, food, toys, medicines, plastic bottles, metal food cans and so on, toxins can lead to cognitive brain dysfunction or thyroid disruption (see RyanDrum.com), learning disorders, ADD, autism and much more. For a list of possible disruptions please see Appendix C.

We have known about environmental contaminants' effects on our health for a very long time yet during the 1918 Great Flu pandemic many physicians continued to use treatments with mercury and arsenic which most likely caused patients to become much sicker.

Yet still this travesty goes unabated. Dr. Alec Pekler, NMD has personal experience with the kind of rigmarole that characterizes righting environmental wrongs. He observes: "It seems that the government and manufacturers downplay the risk of exposure to these toxins. While training as an Environmental Toxicologist, my first degree, I heard a story from one of my professors—the distinguished Dr. John Froines at UCLA. He described how he was testifying on the risks of one of the flame-retardants and urged the government to ban it. The government did ban it but approved another flame-retardant that is almost exactly the same with only a slightly different formula."

It's important to discover your level of toxicity through your integrated primary care physician (iPCP). They can set you up on a protocol that can include chelation. This process detoxifies heavy metal through binding with an agent such as EDTA (I.V. or as a suppository). What you can do at home is get an infrared sauna. This will detox the heavy metals and even plastics like BPA.

HEAVY METALS

The third most abundant mineral on Earth, it is not natural aluminum that is the problem, as this form does not easily absorb through our intestines or our skin. It is rather the manufactured kind. A neurotoxin, it affects the brain through microglia and astrocyte cell activation, disrupts the intestinal epithelium, causes lipid and protein oxidation, and acts as a mitochondrial toxin and damages the kidneys. All that to say, it does not belong in our bodies. (As noted, this has been known this since 1911.[5]) Besides aluminum pots and pans and soda cans and cosmetics, aluminum is in antacids, buffered aspirin, many vaccines, and pharmaceuticals.

Arsenic is another toxin and is in a lot of rice due to the chemical pesticides used in growing cotton in the past. Cadmium is from car batteries, lead is from paint, mercury from dental fillings...the list goes on.

THE ROLE of SULFUR (an ESSENTIAL MINERAL in DETOXIFICATION)[19,20]

Detoxification occurs mainly in the liver where two distinct parts break down toxins, causing oxidation and free radicals (Phase 1) and excrete them (Phase 2).

Phase 1 is activated by pesticides, alcohol, drugs and so on, and in a good way by herbs like *Silybum marianas*, vitamins like C, and cruciferous vegetables, to name a few. Although Phase 1 is helped by the P450 enzyme system it is a dangerous phase because of the potential damaging free radicals. Phase 2 works to get these degrading toxins out through bile, urine and stool by six different pathways, and these must be supported.

One mineral that plays an extremely important role in this is sulfur. Without it the body does not have the necessary tools to get the toxins out.

Sulfur is essential to making methionine and cysteine, two amino acids that involve the production of glutathione, the major antioxidant in the body. Methionine acts as a precursor to SAM—S-adenosylmethionine, a major anti-inflammatory; and cysteine is the precursor to glutathione and then there's taurine, a storage form of sulfur.

Sulfur amino acids are sensitive to ROS (reactive oxygen species), potentially harmful free radicals that damage cells and tissues. The sulfur bound amino acids can attach to ROS, reducing the possibility of oxidative damage (including cell-signaling impairment that can be important in cytokine function.)

One way to get your necessary sulfur is through food: garlic, onions and the sulforaphane compounds found in cruciferous vegetables such as broccoli, cauliflower, cabbage, and other foods (see Nutrition section).

METHYLATION

This metabolic process underscores the problem of deficiency in a mineral like sulfur as the consequences can be dire in the detoxification phases and can affect production and recycling of glutathione, our body's major antioxidant.

Methylation uses methionine from sulfur in a process that attaches a methyl group (one carbon and three hydrogens) to another molecule. Demethylation is the opposite: it removes a methyl group. The problem can lie in our genetics. The MTHFR genetic polymorphisms (meaning there are several manifestations of this gene, *i.e.* homozygous, heterozygous, you can look those up on the internet!) can create an imbalance in this cycle of methylation by inhibiting the conversion of homocysteine, an intermediary metabolite that is implicated in disease.

Methylation supplements, if you need them, support the methylation process, and include choline and the B Vitamins, especially methyl folate and methyl B 12.

THE PROCESS OF DETOXIFICATION

Bile acids, a major pathway of elimination of toxic compounds, conjugate to either taurine or glycine (another amino acid) after being sulfated and then shipped out by the liver. Bifidobacterium in the gut alter bile acids by deconjugating taurine and glycine from bile acid to increase gelling potential. This helps bacteria to colonize the GI tract. eNOS, a cytochrome P450 (CYP) liver enzyme, essential for many metabolic processes including detoxification and nitric oxide release (NO) is vulnerable to toxins such as mercury and aluminum.

The glymphatic system is a waste clearance system for the brain. The 16th century philosopher and scientist, Rene Descartes, called the pineal gland "the seat of the soul" while scientists today regard it as a secreting endocrine gland that produces sulfate by day and then supplies the brain at night with it. Like lymph to the rest of the body, it allows the brain to detox at night and is why it is essential to get a good night's sleep.

Although cholesterol sulfate synthesis in skin after sun exposure gives a good amount of cholesterol and sulfate to the tissues and cells, environmental toxins such as heavy metals and pesticides diminish sulfur in blood. This can lead to an increased susceptibility of infection and other disease due to impaired cholesterol sulfate synthesis.[2, 19]

MIT scientists, Anthony Samsel and Stephanie Seneff,[20] show how interference with CYP (liver) enzymes acts synergistically with disruption of the biosynthesis of aromatic amino acids by gut bacteria, as well as impairment in serum sulfate transport." Consequences are most of the diseases and conditions associated with a Western diet, which include gastrointestinal disorders including celiac disease, obesity, diabetes, heart disease, depression, autism, infertility, cancer and Alzheimer's disease.[18]

Sulfur metabolism is greatly diminished by glyphosate, the ubiquitous and pervasive herbicide, (RoundUp®) according to research. Used to control weeds, these are the raw components of biofuels.[2, 21] Hence we may be contaminated further on highways or in the air. According to a theory put forward by Seneff, it may just be this that is causing extreme damage to the lungs in the same way as E-cigarettes can, compromising the innate immune system. Fatty liver disease has been "rising alarmingly in the population, in step with the rapid rise of glyphosate on core crops over the past two decades." And liver disease is one of the preconditions to a fatal response to the virus in COVID-19.

According to Seneff and other scientists, glyphosate not only disrupts the essential sulfate synthesis and transport, but it disrupts the microbiome of the gut, inhibits liver enzymes of detoxification—P450, impairs methylation processes, chelates important minerals and inhibits the production of TSH, thyroid stimulating hormone.

With insufficient sulfate leading to hypertension and severe bloodclotting, what are your thoughts on this in relation to COVID-19? Yes, the need for sunshine and detoxification, daily!

So how at risk are those in nursing homes? At the slim chance they venture outside they will be slathered with sunscreen (usually toxic) that blocks sulfur (and Vitamin D) from being absorbed.

Therefore, taking time to be in the sunshine, eating foods rich in sulforaphane as well also polyphenols and flavonoids (transporters of sulfate), avoiding environmental toxins and doing a daily detox with an infrared sauna is not just a suggestion.

Now on to a subject most certainly to ruffle a few feathers.

THE TOXICITY OF VACCINES

The problem with vaccines is that they contain substances that interfere with cell function as well as promote inflammation, both affecting the intracellular matrix and the subsequent inability of the cell to detox. The adjuvants, put there to stimulate the immune response and create antibodies, do not involve the Th1 cell mediated side of the immune system, which will clear toxins. Our innate immune system may come to the rescue but not as rapidly or as thoroughly. Thus, these toxins stick around and may cross the blood brain border causing irreparable harm.[15]

Let's look at a common flu vaccine, Fluviron®, that contains the following:[22]

- Thimerosal: a potent neurotoxin that contains mercury,[11] an antibacterial used in multi-dose vials although single doses have it from the original formulation.
- Formaldehyde: a known toxin.
- Beta-propiolactone: extreme toxicity through inhalation in animals; possible carcinogen according to epa.gov.

- Egg protein: Eggs are a very common allergy; injecting egg protein into children can sensitize them to an allergy for life.
- Neomycin: antibiotic.
- Polymyxin B: antibiotic.
- Gentamicin sulfate: antibiotic.
- Hydrocortisone: steroid.
- Polyoxyethylene 9-10 nonyl phenol (triton N-101, octoxynol 9): detergent, extremely toxic to aquatic life.
- Polysorbate-80: detergent; crosses the blood brain barrier.
- Sodium deoxycholate: detergent

MERCURY

You may know mercury from dental amalgams. This is ethyl mercury, continuing to be used in dentistry. (Methylmercury is the contaminant in fish.) Added to prevent bacterial growth in a flu vaccine and called thimerosal, is toxic because mercury is toxic in any state and can cause neuronal deterioration in the central nervous system. Although technically taken out of most single use vaccines it is still in the multi dose and, used in creating the vaccine, with a trace level remaining in the single dose. The FDA says mercury is not safe on skin and in 1998 it barred topical preparations with mercury. If mercury is spilled on a lab floor a Hazmat team must be brought in. Therefore, to say flu shots are safe for pregnant women and children is incorrect. Any form of mercury is toxic.[15,16,17, 23, 24]

The problem with a vaccine, touted in allopathic medicine as a cure-all or prevent-all, coupled with a reverence far beyond its actual capabilities, is the addition of adjuvants or additives to make them more "efficient," as we saw in Fluviron®. These are poisonous and cause the immune system to be chronically over-stimulated, leading to autoimmune diseases such as lupus, rheumatoid arthritis, scleroderma and so on manifesting in fatigue, muscle and neurological difficulties.[24] One study (Vaccine, 2017) found that the risk of miscarriage increased significantly with the vaccination for H1N1 strain.

Vaccination was an interesting idea 100 or so years ago but it's based on old science, not with the knowledge we have of our immune system today. And like environmental toxins, they have had far too little testing for safety and elicit far too many injuries including neurological damage like seizures, autism and even death.

As Thomas Cowan MD writes,[25] "Modern pediatrics is essentially an assault on the cell-mediated immune system...As a public health strategy, (vaccination) leaves a lot of unanswered questions. (Because for one) if you inject a child with a toxin to provoke an antibody response and at the same time suppress the cell-mediated response with acetaminophen, how will the body clear the toxin?"

And what about other vaccines with toxic adjuvants? According to research it may set the child up for having an autoimmune disease.[24] This is evident in the new syndrome ASIA that stands for not the continent but Autoimmunity/Inflammatory Syndrome Induced by Adjuvants.

One consequence in Finland after vaccination for H1N1 (swine flu) was a 13-fold increase in narcolepsy, now considered an autoimmune disease, affecting people with the (HLA) DQB1*0602 genotype. This is an example of a personal or geographic risk but since we don't know which vaccine affects what population best to stay away.

Consider the words of the celebrated Immunologist, on an expert advisory panel on immunology for WHO for twenty years, Hugh Fudenberg, MD. At the International Vaccine Conference in Arlington, VA in 1997 he said that the incidence of Alzheimer Disease is much higher if someone repeatedly has a flu shot; he noted the gradual buildup of mercury and aluminum in the brain causes cognitive dysfunction.

And once again, MIT scientist, Dr. Stephanie Seneff: "The whole (vaccine) system is geared on anti-life. You vaccinate to kill off all the microbes that might infect your body, you know, and then you take all these drugs which are interfering with life in the sense that they're disrupting some enzyme somewhere that's probably very critical to a whole bunch of different functions. The whole thing is just interfering with life. It's such a strange model."[20]

E. Harold Buttram MD wrote[26]: "Bypassing the cellular immune system, current injectable vaccines are directed toward stimulating the humoral system, thus establishing it in relative dominance over the cellular system, the reverse of the natural immunologic scheme that humans evolved with. Childhood vaccine programs may be turning childhood immune systems inside out, with the humoral system being thrown into a dominant position for which it is physiologically unsuited, while cellular immunity, lacking the challenges of the minor childhood diseases of former times, may undergo progressive atrophy from disuse."

We need our old childhood diseases to challenge our immune response. Nature has designed something quite miraculous and by experiencing these early illnesses—utilizing both the cellular and humoral activity that act together to destroy and rid the body of foreign microorganisms from the blood—we benefit from lifelong immunity. This maturation of the immune system means it is better able to fight off chronic diseases and cancer later in life.

Richard Moskowitz in his book, *Vaccines, A Reappraisal,* continues this thought: "Bypassing the normal portal of entry, (the vaccine) gives the live virus, bacterium or adjuvanted fragments free access to the blood and internal organs, where it is designed to remain on a chronic basis, and indeed more or less permanently, thus quite possibly inhibiting the immune system from responding acutely, vigorously and effectively to other invading organism and foreign antigens in the future."

On January 16, 2015 the CBC News posted that the B.C. Centre for Disease Control had discovered "people who receive flu vaccines year after year can sometimes show reduced protection, an effect that Canadian infectious disease specialists say muddies health messages for annual flu vaccine campaigns. This came out when during the 2009 H1N1 pandemic, seasonal flu shots from 2008 were given to protect against the pandemic strain. This in fact doubled the risk of infection from the pandemic flu. The vaccine may weaken an immune system predisposing the person to other infections; thus, in a catch 22 scenario predisposing the person to the flu infection itself." And why did this take six years to be made public is my question.

A tremendous amount of money and mythology and poison goes into vaccine manufacture with nary a word about environmental toxins, increasing access to fresh organic fruits and vegetables for essential vitamins and minerals or learning about inexpensive medicinal plants and homeopathic medicines.

ASSIGNMENT #6

1. What do environmental toxins mean to you? Name three groups.
2. What is the role of sulfur in detoxification? List three of its activities.
3. What is methylation?
4. How can vaccines be harmful?

CHAPTER 7: COVID-19 – Check podcast Dr. Heather Uncensored for any major updates

The Great Flu of 1918-19 had three waves to it. People would get sick for a few months then it would die away for a few months and then it would come back, often more virulent. The US is currently experiencing a second wave, therefore it's important we don't jump to too many conclusions at this point. That said, we need as much information on prevention and natural treatment as we can gather at this stage. The fact that initial assumptions about the way the virus enters *i.e.,* ACE2 host receptor and causes harm are seemingly being proven incorrect as the receptor may in fact be CD147 demonstrates how little is known about this pathogen as of summer 2020.[1,2,3] And that it may be caused by a consequence of toxic contaminants is another factor and just a theory at this point. One thing we do know is that the United States has the highest number of cases and mortality rates as of July 2020. Therefore, please excuse the nature of this chapter: I am simply throwing out ideas that must be considered.

WHERE IT CAME FROM

By now most people probably know a lot about the novel COVID-19 that has disrupted our lives for the last several months during 2020. From a vast family of human coronaviruses (HCoVs) first identified in the Netherlands in the late 1960s and named for its crown-like appearance under a microscope, there are only seven coronaviruses that infect humans. For centuries all these viruses caused was a mild respiratory disease akin to the common cold. It wasn't until the 21st century that scientists discovered these could be harbored in animals and transmitted to humans, and so all cases are zoonotic with the bat being the most likely original source.

A relative to SARS (severe acute respiratory syndrome) with very distinct differences, and MERS (middle eastern respiratory syndrome), and named SARS-CoV-2, the COVID-19 virus has a wide range of symptomatology from mild to severe. Initial diagnosis revealed COVID-19 is clinically milder than SARS that infected 8,000 people with 800 dead (10% mortality rate), the source also most likely coming from a bat, then a civet cat before infecting humans. Currently there are no cases of SARS, but MERS, presumably also initially due to a bat, was first detected in Saudi Arabia in a man's sputum and from a camel, and is still around, although with sporadic cases. Its mortality rate, totaling 30% confirmed with 2,465 cases is significantly higher than that of SARS.[1]

From all reported sources, COVID-19 first reared its ugly head in China's Wuhan province in late December 2019. A wet market that sold live animals including an infected bat believed to be the source of the viral infection, the present COVID-19 pandemic that caused a cluster of pneumonia cases.

At this time, summer 2020, mortality from COVID-19 has far surpassed a bad seasonal flu with over 500,000 deaths reported globally and the numbers continue to climb. However, this is far less than the 50 million from the Great Flu of 1918. While the death toll has passed 150,000 in the US, the mortality rate, as of July 2020, hovers around less than 1%, significantly lower in comparison to previous coronavirus infections.[2] And it is affecting far more Latinx as well as Blacks. This is one question we must answer.

PRESENTATION

The heart wrenching stories of patients who have contracted the COVID-19 virus are escalating as I write this summer of 2020 with many intensive care units once again faced with the ignominious prospect of being overwhelmed with people at a high risk of dying if there exists a comorbidity, most commonly hypertension, then diabetes, and COPD.[1,2,4,5]

Symptoms range from mild to severe or none at all and include fever, dry cough, aches and pains (diffuse myalgia) and fatigue. Headache, increased mucus, and diarrhea may be present but much less so. Approximately half infected will develop shortness of breath (dyspnea) and have lymphopenia (diminished lymphocyte count).[1,2]

In both young and older adults, bilateral interstitial pneumonia can be a serious complication of COVID-19. As it progresses, more of the air sacs, filled with fluid, leak from tiny blood vessels in the lungs that can progress to scarring of lung tissue leading to ARDS (acute respiratory distress syndrome) or ALI (acute lung injury).[1]

Another possible complication is sepsis, meaning the viral infection has reached the bloodstream and causes damage wherever it can get to and can initiate a cytokine storm. Impacting the lungs and the heart can lead to a possible death sentence or likelihood for lasting lung injury.

Respiratory problems are often initially alerted by heart symptoms so keep that in mind if you are caring for someone. In any case, get to the ER asap. Ventilators are not being used to the extent they were at the beginning of the COVID crisis as it meant an almost sure death sentence or long-lasting disability.

TRANSMISSION

The virus was first thought to be transmitted by respiratory droplets from coughing and/or sneezing, that could span up to twenty feet.[2] It now seems it can be aerosolized (transmitted through air) as in influenza and that this can last for several hours.[5]

It was also thought that asymptomatic people can transmit the disease and was why it made it even more important to self-isolate, but this idea is being questioned. I have no clinical data either way but asymptomatic spread seems odd. Perhaps it is our inability to be in touch with our bodies.

The widespread and controversial message to wear a facemask has not been clinically verified and may or may not help the spread, but it does lessen people's fears and show respect for the feelings of others. It seems true that the ability for the virus to infect others is made worse when people are close together and is why social distancing is important. Without social distancing each infection causes three others on average (R is the value for reproduction) but many don't spread the disease at all. Hence the value, the dispersion factor (k) which attempts to describe a disease cluster. The lower the k the more transmission comes from a small number of people. At this time, it is thought this number is 1% and that 80% of secondary transmission comes from a small cluster of individuals.[2]

TESTING

Studies show a variation in a CBC (complete blood count).[1] For example, it may be that an initial blood test shows a normal white blood cell count overall although a reduced number of lymphocytes (remember a type of WBC), insufficient but normal red blood cells (RBCs) and a normal platelet count. A few days later the WBCs may increase. As we shall see a breakdown in RBCs creating low oxygen, but normal lung function may be a common presentation,[6] blood count differentials notwithstanding. (Right now nothing is conclusive.)

Radiology: Chest may show pulmonary infiltrates[2,7] of ground-glass or consolidation (usually bilateral).

A real-time reverse transcription-polymerase chain reaction (rRT-PCR) assay has been developed by the CDC to detect this virus for upper and lower respiratory specimens (such as nasopharyngeal or oropharyngeal swabs, bronchoalveolar lavage, sputum, lower respiratory tract aspirate, nasopharyngeal wash/aspirate or nasal aspirate). In the summer of 2020 U.S. hospital doctors and nurses were telling us that it is not adequately available.[2,7] Elon Musk shows the futility of an accurate diagnosis by the PCR test. He had four in one day, two were positive and two negative. Something is very amiss. Not only is it causing untold grief individually, the outcome of alarm over the potential of an inaccurate result is ruining our economy, causing lockdowns, restaurant closures and so on. (More on current conditions on the podcast.) If you want to know where you stand get an antibody test, this will show past infection.

As far as the issues with the COVID vaccines please see my podcast Dr. Heather Uncensored, starting with #33, Dr. Lyn Patrick.

THE RISKS

An RNA virus and therefore mutable, COVID-19 changes structure but not as quickly as HIV or influenza. It is thought there are hundreds of strains with each area or country having its own unique COVID-19 virus.[6]

Older people with an underlying condition are often told, "It's just old age," accepting this as inevitable instead of a condition to be addressed. There are studies showing only a third of those dying in nursing homes is from the virus, the other two-thirds possibly due to loneliness from the visiting and care restrictions. Again, we don't have exact figures yet.

The highest death rate is for patients over 80. Although children have been sick there have been no fatalities for infected COVID-19 children under nine years of age as of July 2020.[4]

The latest news is that people from 15 to 40 comprise the majority of cases testing positive, some mortal. And despite the dearth of medical reporting on natural prevention and treatment, studies are now beginning to show the benefit of Vitamin D[8] to calm a cytokine storm. A huge part of the population is low in Vitamin D. This is true of zinc[9, 10] as well as Vitamin C.[11] Glutathione is also key, as we shall see.[12]

ENTRY POINT OF THE VIRUS

Presenting about ten days after the initial onset of symptoms, ARDS (acute respiratory distress syndrome) or ALI (acute lung injury) was diagnosed as the main consequences of the virus breaching the host cell through the ACE 2 (angiotensin conversion enzyme 2) receptor.[13,14] That is now being questioned and another receptor CD147[6] is up for consideration.

A virus of any kind has a specific way to hijack our cells with unique areas on the host for the virus to breach. In COVID-19, the glycoprotein crown-like spikes called S proteins on the virus protrude hoping to latch onto a receptor in the host cell. If binding occurs it can become activated by the enzyme furin.[6] (specific to this virus) that will cleave the viral envelope and allow the virus to enter the host cells. (Similar to a cytokine, furin can act ambivalently when the body is threatened by infection. Although this protein normally activates many cellular proteins in the body, it can have an aberrant expression. Because furin is present normally in lungs as well as the liver and small intestine, the virus can potentially attack several organs at once.) This snipping allows the amino acid sequences of the host to be exposed and the virus gains access to glycoproteins to assemble and replicate itself.

Also called Basigen or EMMPRIN (extracellular matrix metalloproteinase inducer) CD 147 is a common cell membrane protein known for various physiological and pathological activities.[3] It regulates lymphocyte activity, has significant anti-inflammatory effects[6] and functions as a signaling receptor with cyclophilin A in acute lung inflammation. CyPA that has been identified in viral infections as well as asthma, sepsis and other conditions; together CD147 and CyPA are implicated in kidney disease.[15]

In the beginning doctors assumed the need for a mechanical ventilator due to low arterial oxygen saturation. However, what those in the midst of the battle are now seeing is that abnormal blood clots, embolisms, myocardial infarctions and thrombotic microangiopathy (TMAs = irregular blood clotting events) are developing despite normal lung function.[17] This is further evidence for altering our perspective that COVID-19 is not principally an airflow problem and the need for ventilators has been unwarranted.

TMAs are known to occur in small blood vessels, mostly the kidneys and the brain but the common cause is the usually very rare disease, thrombotic thrombocytopenic purpura (TTP) where platelets clump together to form minute blood clots in small vessels. TMAs can also be caused by aHUS, atypical hemolytic uremic syndrome as well as complement activation.[6,16] It seems these TMAs are leading to hemolysis, breakdown of red blood cells.[6] Free heme can cause platelet adhesion and aggregation. This oxidized heme can lead to the NLRP3 inflammasome.[18]

The virus targets heme that dissociates the Fe from porphyrin.[17] This attack leads to less hemoglobin therefore decreasing the amount of oxygen and carbon dioxide which will then distress the respiratory system. Cells in the lung become toxic and inflamed which shows up like ground glass in lung imagery. Now because capillaries have been rendered fragile[19] and easily broken, fibrogen comes in and fills these gaps through coagulation *i.e.* blood clotting.[6] (Diabetics have a risk factor since glycosylated hemoglobin linked to the sugar molecule make RBCs more fragile and increases hemolysis.)

The binding of ACE2 in the host cell is not enough to explain the hypoxemia and heart muscle injury of the abnormal clotting and blockages. ACE2 receptors[6,13,14] are not in blood or bone marrow and do not have furin, known to be high in COVID-19 patients. Furin is used by the CD147-cyclophilin A signaling pathway, highly active including in red blood cells, endothelial cells, cardiomyocytes, lymphocytes as well as platelets.[6,3] Loh has therefore singled out the CD147 receptors on red blood cells,[3,20] hypothesizing that this pathway initiates the damage (oxidative hemolysis yielding excess coagulation, thrombosis and cardiac changes) that ultimately leads to heart failure, and makes the virus up to 1000 times more easily transmissible! (At this point these are theories.)

When the virus binds to the host cell it destroys membranes and increases oxidative stress and results in the activation of the NLRP3 inflammasome that will lead to the deadly cytokine storm primarily through interleukins (cytokines) IL-1B and IL- 18. This NLRP3 inflammasome[18] is key to inducing ARDS/ALI resulting in hypoxia that is induced by IL-1B signaling and dependent on NLRP3 inflammasome.[15] Throughout its pathogenic pathway, Loh postulates the destruction of red blood cells, platelet aggregation, irregular blood clots, thrombosis and finally myocardial injury is an over reactivity that increases the possibility of a cytokine storm leading to possible host cell death and ultimately kidney failure.

MELATONIN TO THE RESCUE

Loh paints a grim picture indeed but her paper also offers a plausible preventive treatment.[6,21,20] In hemolysis and blood clotting, oxygen does not get to where it needs to be to keep us well and alive. These red blood cells are fragile and misshapen and in desperate need of antioxidants. Loh's answer to this is the "ancient pleiotropic molecule,"[6] melatonin, ubiquitous and abundantly available in children. Used to protect red blood cells from oxidative hemolysis (being damaged and broken down), melatonin can "reverse hemolytic anemia, normalize heme synthesis, restore lymphocytes and platelet counts, and reduce vessel permeability during an acute hemolytic crisis by maintaining intracellular calcium homeostasis and reduction of oxidative stress."[6]

Melatonin, according to various sources[6,20] can inhibit NLRP3 inflammasomes, dramatically reducing pulmonary injury, as well as decreasing infiltration of macrophages and neutrophils into the lungs. This translates into much less infection with the resulting ARDS or ALI.[17]

That children have very high melatonin is believed to be the reason there have been no fatalities in children under nine years of age. Pregnant mothers also benefit from high melatonin secretion in the third trimester, double that of the first semester, which possibly explains why pregnant women are not dying from COVID-19.[17]

Another factor that serves the melatonin hypothesis is that melatonin is known to increase the production of glutathione,[12] which with Vitamin C, constitute the most abundant antioxidants in the body and hence increase fibrinolysis or fibrin breakdown, the basis of clots. Since glutathione, Vitamin C and melatonin can inhibit platelet activation and normalize platelet counts in people with thrombocytopenia,[11] we can add them along with melatonin to our list of suggested supplements.

One last substance we can manipulate is nitric oxide (NO).[9,18,22] This inhibits the NLRP3 inflammasome,[9,18] reduces oxidative stress, furin expression, regulates hypoxia signaling, mitochondrial function and modulates other immune defenses to lessen the consequence of a cytokine storm.[6,9,18] Another great quality in terms of fighting a viral infection is that NO is produced in the nasal passages as part of the immune system's first defense.[15,23] (Dosages are in Part 4.)

Dr. Seneff's recent paper about glyphosate[24] and its connection in COVID-19 is presented in the chapter, *The Burden of Environmental Toxins*. This is a scenario that is truly devastating and forces everyone to consider organic food as a societal essential.

We are at a grim crossroads here in America with respect to how we care for the sick and the apparently well. In light of the abundance of nursing home deaths it seems poor nutrition likely coupled with clogged lymph and poor detoxification including the current standard of a pill for every ailment, represents the cause for such a disastrous consequence of this current virus. The other, now apparent glaring omission of care has surfaced from the fact that African Americans[25] and Latinx are succumbing at a much higher rate than Caucasians. One factor is that 82% of blacks are deficient in Vitamin D (melanin blocks absorption) compared to 40% of the white population and we know that Vitamin D deficiency may be the most important factor in your immune system overreacting and creating a cytokine storm. (Therefore, to recommend 10-20 minutes a day of midday sun to people of color is inadequate.)

It seems COVID-19 has highlighted not only the danger of consuming what is known as the standard North American Diet (SAD), a diet of low nutritional status and replete with toxic particles including the very dangerous glyphosate from the weed killer RoundUp® but racial bias.

TREATMENT

From the foregoing research we can speculate that melatonin, Vitamin C, Vitamin D, and zinc are the most important in supplementation and a daily detox to outwit COVID-19. And as we shall see evidence of positive results, whether prophylactically or during treatment, is piling up for Homeopathy, botanical medicine is showing promise from including the much-loved antiviral *Glycyrrhiza glabra* and as important the need to get into the sunshine - to absorb not just the cytokine quieter Vitamin D but to activate sulfur, the mineral so necessary for detoxification. (It's not always about what you consciously put into your body but what you can get out. If at all possible, invest in an infrared sauna). (See Resources)

As a final thought, for those lucky enough to have repelled a serious attack of COVID-19 and survived, there is ample evidence to indicate debilitating fatigue may follow and can last for months. Please see the last chapter in this book, The Aftermath.

Meanwhile eat well, organic only, take the minimum of of melatonin, Vitamin C, D and zinc and implement a daily detox.

COVID-19 VACCINE

SARS-CoV-2 (COVID-19) is an mRNA virus, which means it mutates (as discussed). New strains are coming into the US from England and Nigeria of late. As of early 2021 a large percentage of frontline health workers are refusing the vaccine. Thank goodness. It makes no sense to add toxic substances, the adjuvants of a vaccine added to make it more "efficient" when we are already compromised by our polluted world. There have been so many side effects. The latest statistic was a 94 year old woman who died within four-hours of receiving the vaccine. If you get it at this time you are agreeing to be a guinea pig as there have been virtually no clinical trials. It's your choice but please do the research.

For updates to this chapter and vaccine ingredients from the various pharmaceutical companies, please listen to the podcast "*Dr. Heather Uncensored.*"

ASSIGNMENT #7

1. How does SARS-COV-2 breach a host cell? Include receptor sites that have been theorized.
2. How may melatonin and Vitamin C help thwart the COVID-19 virus?
3. What is glyphosate and how is it dangerous?
4. Why is a daily detox important?

PART THREE: NATUROPATHIC MEDICINE

PRESENT DAY

There are several currently license-able systems of medicine that are holistic, integrative, that stay true to nature's hand in healing. These are naturopathic medicine, Traditional Chinese Medicine including acupuncture, osteopathic medicine, and chiropractic medicine. Unfortunately, at this time homeopathic medicine and botanical medicine are not licensable on their own and are practiced within one of these systems.

There are seven naturopathic medical schools in North America: Bastyr: Seattle and San Diego Campuses, Boucher Institute of Naturopathic Medicine, Vancouver, BC, National University of Natural Medicine, Portland, OR, Southwest College of Naturopathic Medicine and Health Sciences, Phoenix, AZ, The Canadian College of Naturopathic Medicine, Toronto, ON and the National University of Health Sciences, Chicago, IL.

As we shall see in the next chapter, physicists are only now beginning to understand the relevance of the vital force and that it jives with the theories of matter and energy in the field of physics, namely quantum field theories.

BACKGROUND

Naturopathic Medicine arose from other medical systems in the late 1800s: Nature Cure which believes in the essential benefits of fresh air, sunshine, exercise, clean water and food, Eclectic medicine that added botanicals, and Homeopathy, an energetic medicine of which physicists are now taking note. Both are based on the philosophy of Vitalism and the motto vis *medicatrix naturae,* the healing power of nature. This concept means that all living beings possess a vital energy giving us an innate ability to heal. This energy is called the vital force in Naturopathic Medicine and refers to the inherent wisdom of the body, that it is always working toward healing, if given the right conditions.

Vitalistic philosophy (and healing) dates back to Greece and Hippocrates. Known as the father of modern medicine Hippocrates was influenced by TCM and Ayurvedic philosophies and practices. Much literature of this, including ancient texts, was lost when libraries were burned during the Dark Ages in Europe.

It turns out that most traditional cultures around the world have a name for this vitalistic energy with almost 100 different names. For instance, Ayurvedic Medicine with its roots in India refers to it as prana while Traditional Chinese Medicine (TCM) calls it qi. Relying on a holistic model we eat well, drink clean water, utilize botanicals to boost our host response, homeopathy to boost our vital force or "qi", and use hydrotherapy to increase circulation and lymph maximizing oxygen to the tissues and ensuring efficient waste removal. These methods bolster our innate and adaptive immune systems in both prevention status and in the sick room when a dangerous virus like influenza or COVID-19 has breached our cells.

CHAPTER 8: HOMEOPATHIC MEDICINE - "NANO-PEARLS"

When I began this book I could never, in my wildest dreams, have imagined that I would be attending a conference where the first slide of the keynote speaker, a Nobel Prize winner in physiology, would read: Homeopathy is the future of science and medicine.

But this is exactly what happened at JAHC2020, a global homeopathic summit held in June 2020. Dr. Luc Montagnier, who discovered HIV, the cause of AIDS, went on to say that his physicist friends had done a study of homeopathic dilutions and saw what they call a "chain of nano-pearls." (In the International System of Units, a "nano" is one-billionth of a meter - a sheet of paper 100,000 nanometers thick gives you an idea.)

Despite the dark cloud of COVID-19 hovering over our heads, here at last was homeopathy validated by science. Ah, the bliss of it. At last. And then, inducing another wave of ecstasy, Dr. Montagnier announced that aluminum, in most vaccines, is very harmful. He showed slides of sheep being affected by this neurotoxin.

Homeopaths from all backgrounds and allies showed up from around the world to learn and share. Presentations included homeopathic research, case studies, the novel German homeopathic research project of Reishi mushroom that is being considered by the author, Ana Schade, a remedy for our time, ongoing homeopathic AIDS clinics in Africa with Jeremy and Camilla Scherr, the mention of the US Sidewalk Clinic, and so much more.

For someone with a deep love of homeopathy it was a conference of a lifetime, a time when after decades of ridicule "we are," as New York homeopath and educator, Denise Staiges, laughed, "the cool kids on the block."

ENERGY MEDICINE

Homeopathy is an energetic medicine based on serial dilutions of a substance including safe or toxic plants, bodily secretions, or toxic chemicals. It has been practiced all over the world since its discovery in the 1700s and has had tremendous success in treating epidemics and pandemics, outpacing allopathic at everyone.[1,2,3,4]

As well, prophylactic (preventive) homeopathic medicine has been shown to be extraordinarily effective in the past and the present in countries such as India, Cuba, and Kenya. This is especially noteworthy as generating protection from a disease for a global population at a low cost is essential.

Homeopathy gets a bad rap especially in the United States because this country is so materially focused. What a shame considering homeopathy's history of surpassing orthodox or allopathic physicians in epidemics. As an example, in 1934, Dr. W.A. Pearson, Dean of the Hahnemann Medical College of Philadelphia, reported that in their hospital of 592 beds, "he carefully collected records of 26,795 cases of epidemic flu, including 1918, treated by homeopathic physicians, with the low mortality rate of practically 1 percent, whilst for the same epidemics the Orthodox rate was 30 percent." (Aspirin and Quinine were the drugs of choice of the allopaths and apparently no homeopath lost a case unless the patient was first dosed with aspirin.[5])

Dr. Joel Shepperd wrote a paper entitled *Hahnemann's Pure Method of Science* underscoring Hahnemann's integrity and intelligence: his "works are the result of careful observation of phenomena, rigorous experimentation, and repeatable verifications. In other words, he has created a science... He developed a purely descriptive method of science rather than a theoretical science... None of his conclusions are based on theories."[6]

HISTORY

The principle of homeopathy, "like cures like", can be traced back to the Greek physician, Hippocrates (460-377 BCE) but its practice that led to a system is due to Dr. Samuel Hahnemann, an Austrian medical doctor who made house calls by horse and buggy in the 1700s. He observed that after a day of his herbal preparations bouncing along beside him that these had a more positive action on his patients than earlier in the day. Over time he also observed that the least amount of medicine from these herbs the better the effect.

He studied these plant tinctures systematically, noted their effects on healthy subjects before experimenting with dilution to the point the medicine contained no molecules, only its energetic layer - the chain of nano-pearls - that he found to help the sick immensely, including the mentally ill, although he didn't make this distinction, instead seeing the whole person.

In 1792 the Duke of Saxe-Gotha conferred the charge of an asylum for the insane where Hahnemann proclaimed publicly that he proposed to adopt "gentle methods."[2]

At this point in history, the mentally ill were normally put in dungeons, chained, and whipped. Thankfully Hahnemann saw another way: "I never allow an insane person to be punished, either by blows or any kind of corporeal chastisement...these sufferers only deserve pity and are always worse after such rough and cruel treatment."[2] He also opposed the large and repeated doses of nauseating medicines that these inmates were forced to swallow.

Within a year of being in charge of the Gotha asylum, Hahnemann was able to cure the Secretary of the Chancellery of Hanover, Herr Klockenbring who had been treated for insanity - "eccentricities, delusions, and a tendency to destroy his clothing, the furniture, piano."[6] Previously, the Hanoverian court physician, Herr Dr. Wichmann, had treated Klockenberg without success. Of further note in 1799, during an epidemic of scarlet fever Hahnemann discovered that Belladonna can be used prophylactically.[2,7] (This is a topic we will cover later.)

Calling attention to another historic figure, Dr. Henry Holcombe M.D. was a successful physician who practiced in the 19th century in Louisiana. A convert from allopathy to homeopathy he had tremendous success in the yellow fever epidemics, writing: "When one has grasped the idea that by creative laws mind (thought) is dormant in all things of the body, the minutest changes of which are in reality organic manifestations or showing forth of mental conditions, many things before incomprehensible become clear. From the standpoint of this grand truth we see how emotions (which are produced by thought) determine the most rapid changes in the secretions of our body; how fright turns the hair gray; how terror poisons the mother's milk; how great mental excitements or the slow torture of mental anxiety write their baneful effects upon the tissues of the brain;..."[7] He continues a few paragraphs later, "The part which the mind has always played in the cure has been ignored, or not recognized, because of the prevalent and dominant spirit of materialism. The mind (thought) has been all the time counted out, while in reality it may have been the chief and perhaps the only factor in the case. When we are confronted with cures of the most remarkable character, cures entirely beyond the reach of our best medication, we attribute them to imagination, faith, hope, expectations. And we do so rightly; for imagination, faith, hope, expectation are states of mind, are the mind itself in substantial activity and creativity energy, and when these vital forces can be evoked and directed there is no limit to the possibilities that lie in store for us."[7]

Again, the New Thought Movement influence: thought can make you sick or it can make you well...

Ethelbert Petrie Hoyle, M.D. (1861-1955) a British orthodox physician who also converted to homeopathy and contributed to our wealth of historical knowledge, wrote: "One great difference between the two schools of medicine is that orthodoxy is always flirting with the 'maximum' dose ...We homeopaths always aim at giving the most minute medical stimulus, never harmful, which will arouse the vital reaction towards natural repair, and we have a guiding rule *(similia)* on which to base every prescription."[5] (As an aside, Petrie Hoyle lived in San Francisco periodically between 1895 to 1910.)

None other than Albert Einstein, PhD, famously said, "There is a particle and a wave to everything."[8] Homeopathy is the wave that has been captured on "seeds," as my young patients called them. This explanation appeases people who have depended on the material doses of allopathy for a long time but are hoping to make the switch to something more natural.

And now Dr. Luc Montaignier, and others after almost 250 years, Hahnemann's observation and intuition is being verified.

MORTALITY RATES

Mortality rates during epidemics in the 19th and 20th century differ so widely between the two medical systems. According to Thomas Lindsley Bradford M.D.'s book published in 1900 by Boerke and Tafel, *The Logic of Figures or Comparative Results of Homeopathic and Other Treatments*, shows that 1813, a typhus fever outbreak in the wake of Napoleon's retreat in Germany, Hahnemann lost only two patients of 180, less than 1% while the allopaths lost over 30%. Cholera, 1831 in Austria and 1854 in London, showed similar successes with homeopathic treatment.

Consider 1854 when cholera hit London, finally sourced to a polluted public water pump. Under allopathic care the mortality rate was 59% while under homeopathic care 9%, which as a naturopathic medical doctor I find doubling interesting as homeopathy was able to address the symptoms generated by a polluted water pump. (Many books have been written about the fact homeopathic data was withheld at first in the assessment of mortality rates and what was working in order not to skew the numbers!)

Henry Holcombe M.D. in New Orleans gathered statistics from the devastating yellow fever epidemics in the mid-1800s that occurred there on a regular basis due to the port - ships coming in from the Caribbean of Africa. In fact, this was one reason slavery ended since it prevented ships from entering port!! Holcombe noted a mortality rate with homeopathy of 0.7% (no pneumonia) and 3.4% (with pneumonia) or while conventional or allopathic rates averaged 6% to 30% (even 50%!)[9]. His book, *Yellow Fever and its Homeopathic Treatment* from 1856, is available as is the 1860 book by C. Neidhard, *The Efficacy of Crotalus Horridus in Yellow Fever.*

One homeopathic researcher, Dr. Lisa Samet, found the chances of surviving with homeopathy overall to be 148 to 1 while the conventional route knocked it down to 16 to 1. That is over eight times higher, and if pregnant, your chances jumped 41 times more likely to die![10,11]

Dr S.H. Grimmer of Chicago was reported to say, "It is a rare thing for pneumonia to develop if a good homeopathic physician is called during the first 24 hours of an attack of influenza."

Close to 1.5 million children worldwide die every year from pneumonia, more than AIDS, malaria and TB combined. It is the leading cause of death from infectious diseases in the United States, killing with a secondary, bacterial, pathogen. These alarming statistics are due to, as with many diseases, a resistance to antibiotics. Isn't it time to spread the word of homeopathy's successes, allowing it to inform public health policy? Not only is it effective, it is inexpensive and non-toxic, something the world can use with a high level of confidence as reflected in statistical data.

As clinical researcher Dr. Andre Saine, debating skeptic Dr. Steven Novella at the University School of Medicine in 2013, said, "Homeopathy offers the safest and best outcomes ever demonstrated by any system of medicine for patients with pneumonia and therefore would receive the highest possible recommendations of any intervention for these patients."

The substantial literature on homeopathy during epidemics and pandemics compare allopathic and homeopathic mortality rates. With more than 9,000 references with 500 books and pamphlets to draw from, the facts are clear: homeopathy has a much lower mortality rate no matter how high the mortality rate of the disease, who the physician is, or the time or place, while taking modern nursing and hygiene into account.

In some cases, a homeopathic medicine that fit the symptoms was used while other times a nosode, a homeopathic medicine made from the disease itself is or was used.

HOMEOPATHIC PROPHYLAXIS FOR DISEASE PREVENTION

The varying cost of a physician aside, using homeopathy as prevention can be an extremely inexpensive way to cover a population that is at danger of a viral or bacterial epidemic. Consider Brazil in 1974-75 with an epidemic of meningococcal meningitis (*Neisseria meningitidis*) that spread through overcrowded slums, killing 80% of the population. (No antibiotics.) However, when in Guaratingueta, a city in the state of Sao Paulo, children received the homeopathic medicine "Meningococcinum A and C" as prophylaxis, the control group (no homeopathic medicine) contracted the disease seven times more. Other examples include India, in the state of Uttar Pradesh, in 1991, with Japanese encephalitis (mortality rate 30%) using Belladonna prophylactically with follow ups showing no cases of the illness. In the book, *Homeopathy Heals,* Louise McLean notes that Dr. Francisco Eizayaga of Argentina talked about a polio epidemic in Buenos Aires in 1957 in which thousands of doses of *Lathyrus sativa* 30c were distributed and nobody suffered. In Cuba, in 2007 and 2008, an annual epidemic of Leptospirosis, a tropical disease transmitted by rats leading to jaundice and kidney failure, researchers discovered an

84% reduction in the disease through the use of a nosode of *Leptospirosis*, homeopathic prophylaxis with the cost of 10% of conventional treatment.

There are many more examples. (Please check out work by *Americans for Homeopathy Choice*, André Saine N.D., Lisa Samet N.D., Jeremy Sherr and more. See Resources.)

UNIQUENESS OF ONE OR THREE MEDICINES IN AN EPIDEMIC = GENUS EPIDEMICUS

Outside of an acute epidemic, case taking for a chronic condition is individualized and there are many, many medicines to choose from. In an epidemic however there is usually only one or a few medicines that will suit the picture of the disease. This was termed *Genus epidemicus* by Hahnemann who observed that any epidemic tends to favor certain homeopathic medicines, underscoring the totality of symptoms (common and peculiar) found in the majority of patients.

Hahnemann's first use of this concept was in a scarlet fever epidemic over two centuries ago where he successfully prescribed Belladonna both prophylactically and for treatment.

In the 19th century in New Orleans during an epidemic of yellow fever, a hemorrhagic fever (blood coming out of orifices), Dr. Holcombe used *Crotalus horridus*, made from rattlesnake, to allay the symptoms and disease.

In the Great Flu of 1918 homeopathic doctors discovered *Bryonia alba, Gelsemium, Eupatorium perfoliatum* and *Rhus Toxicodendron* were the most effective no matter where in the world you contracted the virus. In other epidemics of flu, *Arsenicum album, Baptisia, Influenzinum* as well as *Rhus Toxicodendron,* have been most effective. [6,2]

As of June 2020, there is no consensus of a genus in COVID-19. In fact, in Dr. Paul Herscu's lecture at the global homeopathic summit he spoke about the majority of people (80% with a chronic condition) needing a higher dose of their constitutional medicine or a completely different constitutional medicine. Only in 15% of the group (in normal health) was an acute medicine shown to be appropriate. The remaining 5% would have a terrible response to the virus and would in our world governed by allopathic medicine be put on oxygen or a ventilator. What this says to me, without going into too much detail, is that 80% of the population is so constitutionally sick they can't muster an acute response as the 15% could. Is this due to a poor diet, toxic environment, I can only assume. Research needs to be done. If only 15% of people are able to conjure a reaction to a pathogenic virus that is hijacking their cells it is no wonder the United States has the highest cases and mortality rate than any other country in the world.

APPLICATION IN RESEARCH IN AN EPIDEMIC

There have been different approaches or applications of homeopathic medicine in an epidemic including individualization, *Genus epidemicus*, combination remedies, and isopathy, as reflected in homeopathic research.

The consensus in taking a case individually (individualization) in an epidemic is impracticability: in an urgent global situation the need for timeliness and low cost is paramount. Combination remedies can be effective, according to Jennifer Jacobs M.D.[1,3] if based on a given epidemic in a specific location. Another route is isopathy—similar to vaccinations but on an energetic frequency with no harmful adjuvants - may be attractive to public health because of its similarity to vaccines.

Genus epidemicus has been shown to be highly effective through statistics from research over the last almost two centuries. As Dr. Jacobs said, we need to "refine... and build on the knowledge base with additional rigorous trials."

Lionel R. Milgram, a British chemist and homeopath, has several highly interesting papers discussing homeopathy in terms of quantum entanglement and for our interest, the mode of action of the *Genus epidemicus* during an epidemic.

He created a formula where PPR=patient-practitioner-remedy interaction, Px=patient, Pr=practitioner, and Rx=potentized medicine. Through considering entelechy, the realization of potential (the guiding vital principle of an organism or system), he developed a quantized gyroscopic analogue of the Vital Force=Vf.[12]

With any luck, we will be able to have the rigorous trials Jacobs recommended in the present time but also have more reviews of observations and tallies in the last centuries.[13,4]

DIAGNOSIS - AN EXAMPLE

One example of assessing a current viral illness is given by Paul Herscu ND, MPH. He cites *Gelsemium* (frontal pressure, extreme weakness, exhaustion, etc.) for what seems a common cold, *Mercurius* (intense vomiting, no constipation or diarrhea but chills and sweats, clear to yellow coating on tongue, slight swelling of tongue forming scalloped edges) for a more severe GI viral infection, *i.e.* stomach flu, and *Eupatorium perfoliatum* (muscle aches, headaches, eye pain, sinus congestion, extreme weakness) for a more severe influenza-like illness. Please see Paul's blog of December 31, 2019 for further details.

You might want to get the transcripts for the JAHC2020 and listen to all the possibilities of medicines. Of interest to me because they are different from epidemic expectations: *Antimonium tartaricum* (a very weak state with "rattling of mucus and little expectoration") and Alumina (confusion and constipation). More on this later.

MORE ON HOW TO FIND THE RIGHT REMEDY

First, let's be clear…Hahnemann believed there is something called "obstacles to cure" meaning poor choices in food, destructive emotions, environmental contaminants etc. that all need to be addressed either before or while a homeopathic medicine is given. This is why a naturopathic physician with board certification or substantial training in homeopathy (and is vaccine hesitant) is a good choice as they use a myriad of non-suppressive modalities: clinical nutrition, botanical medicine, psychological framing etc. as well. (Of course many other types of integrated doctors or well-trained homeopaths will understand this too.)

Taking a case in an acute infection is very different from taking a constitutional case. In the latter you sit with someone, listening, asking questions, for two hours (at least in North America), trying to connect the dots that will point to the correct homeopathic medicine, far more than the twenty cited here that are specific for Influenza.

In an acute situation you have a sick person who may not want to speak…so it becomes more about looking, refining your observation skills. What's important is to be open to what the patient is experiencing. If you are taking your own case: consider that the person who has themselves as a patient has a fool for a doctor but sometimes there is no choice.

Once you compile a few symptoms you can check out the keynotes as you familiarize yourself with the homeopathic medicines cited. And check the *Genus epidemicus* if it is known this is in fact an epi or pandemic.

Look for what's unusual if the *Genus epidemicus* isn't having an effect. Are they sweating or having chills at strange times…are they giddy when they should be relaxing, are they unusually tense or afraid…do they want ice in their water…do they not want you to leave them for a second…did they just throw something at you…and then check the keynotes of particular homeopathic medicines.

EVERYONE HAS THEIR OWN WAY OF PRESCRIBING

Some people swear by *Oscillicinum®* at the first sign of flu. At the summit there were a wide range of medicines that were having an effect including: *Tussilago petasites, China officianalis,* the COVID nosode (a homeopathic preparation from the disease component), Camphora, *Tuberculosum iveri,* along with what you'd expect *Gelsemium, Bryonia, Arsenicum album and Eupatorium perfoliatum.*

Prophylactically the COVID-19 nosode is getting a good review. One dose of 1M although there are others who recommend lower potencies. India and Nepal are having good results using low potency *Arsenicum album.*

The other time a homeopathic medicine may be needed is after the illness. Many people will be experiencing tremendous fatigue. Medicines working include *Phosphoric acid, Conium* (worse sex),

Gelsemium (dizzy, headache), *China officinalis* and *China arsenicum.*

TAKING A CASE FOR A NON-HOMEOPATH WHEN NO GENUS EPIDEMICUS IS FORTHCOMING

You can also try this: At the first sign of a chill or any symptom if there is an influenza epidemic, advise them to take a low dose (3x, 6x, 12x or 30x) of *Aconite* alone, alternatively with *Belladonna,* every half hour for five or six doses. Take the pellets straight from the vial. Review in a few hours.

OBSERVE SYMPTOMS

- Body temperature: Fever? Feel hot? Feel Cold? To themselves; to you?
- Thirst: Hot liquids? Cold? Room temperature?
- Pain: location, kind.
- Cough: what time of day, how does it sound?
- Mood: sad, angry, listless.
- Peculiar symptoms: for instance, laughing when very ill.

The particular symptoms must be considered every time...if it isn't quite the simillimum...and a few hours later if you are reconsidering, take the case again with new eyes. It is during this time you can use cool cloths, encourage alkaline water with a straw or in an ice cube...this will not antidote the homeopathic medicine.

HAVE THESE HOMEOPATHIC MEDICINES IN YOUR KIT:

Aconite
Arsenicum album
Baptisia tinctoria
Belladonna
Bryonia alba

Camphora officinarum
Causticum
Chelidonium
COVID-19 nosode
Dulcamara
Eupatorium perfoliatum
Euphrasia officinalis
Ferrum phosphoricum
Gelsemium sempervirens
Influenzinum
Kali bich
Mercurius sol
Nux vomica
Oscillococcinum
Phosphorus
Phytolacca
Pyrogenium
Rhus Toxicodendron
Sulphur
Tussilago (as per Dr Robin Murphy)

- Get a copy of *Boericke's Materia Medica* so you can study each medicine in more detail.

KEYNOTES

- Here is a snapshot to get you started.

Aconite	Aconite is often given during the early phase of respiratory infections. • Deep, phobic situation after fright or shock. • A state of ANGUISH in mind and body. • Physical and mental restlessness. • Sudden and violent symptoms, with fever after exposure to dry, cold weather, cold drafts, also hot weather. • Head bursting, oppressed breathing on least motion. Worse at night and after midnight.
Allium Cepa	• Copious water in eyes, extremely acrid nasal discharge. • (Tears may burn but not excoriate like Euphrasia.) • Better in the open air.
Arsenicum Album	• Difficult to distinguish from Aconite. • Same great anxiety and restlessness. • Felt in pit of stomach. • Very weak. • Needs constant company, thinks will die. • Moans and groans and weeps with fear. • Burning pains anywhere. • And high fever but still chilly. • Worse after midnight to 3 pm. • Similarity to distemper in dogs
Baptisia Tinctoria	• Very toxic state. • Confusion as if drunk. • Delirious. • Falls in and out of deep sleep.

Belladonna	• Heat, redness, throbbing, burning. • Great children's remedy for fever.
Bryonia Alba	• Extremely irritable. • Headache. • Lying perfectly still. • No light. • Intense dryness of all mucous membranes. • May have blood laced mucus. • Lips cracked. • Drinks large quantities of liquids. • Constipated. • Coughing causes sharp pains in throat, chest and head. • Talks business even being so sick. • Worried. • Very tired.
Camphora Officinarum	• State of collapse with icy coldness of the whole body but still wants to throw covers off.
Causticum	• Compulsive anxiety. • Concerned about injustice; very sympathetic. • Hoarse.
Chelidonium	• Reflects liver and gallbladder distress. • Aggressive, domineering, irritable.

Eupatorium Perfoliatum	• Intense pains in the bones, especially long bones. • Flesh feels beaten. • Can't bear the slightest touch. • Fever. • Very restless but tries to contain themselves.
Euphrasia Officinalis	• Indifferent, doesn't want conversation. • Acrid tears and discharge from nose but not excoriating.
Ferrum Phosphoricum	• Another first stage medicine (but with few clear symptoms as an indication). • Easy flushing. • Wants to be alone although can be excited. • Coughing up blood. • High fever. • Pneumonia.
Gelsemium Sempervirens	• Slow onset. • Great weakness. • Dizzy, drowsy, dullness, trembling. • Slow pulse. • Mental apathy, listless.
Influenzi num	• I don't use it; some swear by it.
Mercurius Solubilis	• Salivary secretions increased. • Great thirst. • Terrible breath. • Delirium. • Moans and groans.

Nux Vomica	• Irritable, • Sensitive to noise, light, odors. • Angry when consoled.
Oscillococcinum	• Only at onset. • I don't use it; some swear by it.
Phosphorus	• Wants sympathy. • Very anxious. • Thirsty for cold gulps of water. • Pneumonia.
Pyrogenium (Similar To Baptisia)	• Great for septic states. • All discharges offensive. • A lot of pain. • High pulse but not that high a fever.
Rhus Toxicodendron	• Helpless, crying. • Extreme restlessness, constantly trying to change position. • Triangular red tip on tongue, the rest coated and dry. • Can be spitting or coughing up frank blood.
Sulphur	• Always thinks he knows what's best for him/her. • Thirsty for ice cold. • Doesn't want to wash.

Veratrum Viride	• Intense fever with very foul breath. • Narrow red streak down center of tongue. • Twitching and convulsions. • Blood pressure falling. • Pneumonia with increased pulse.

FINAL NOTES

If you are not a homeopath it's important to take classes. It is not an easy study but studying to be prepared during a pandemic like COVID-19 is an excellent opportunity to understand the potential of homeopathy. The bottom line is that homeopathic medicine nudges the body's healing energy (also called qi, vital force) that can be hustled or spun into action but you have to be an excellent observer to match the medicine with the person's state of disease.

Like other modalities used by naturopathic or integrated physicians to help relieve the stress of a virus, homeopathy seeks to assist rather than suppress the body's power to heal. In this way it is not the virus one is concerned with but rather the body's immune system, its defense system, the way it responds to the invader that is important. And it depends what the individual's weaknesses are, how the body tries to return to health, to normalcy.

It's not the fever or coughing or headache or diarrhea or the emotional or mental state but it is the observation of the whole picture…what makes it unique or peculiar. In a super influenza or other epidemic/pandemic there can be a *Genus epidemicus* and this is what makes treating it different in a viral infection affecting many people. Once the genus is known it can be a bit simpler to know what to give. I urge you to read the writings on epidemics and pandemics including statistics of Lisa Samet, ND, Andre Saine, ND, and Robin Murphy, ND, my first homeopathic teacher, Monday evenings at Bastyr in 1983. Others include Lisa Amerine, ND, Jeremy Scherr and so many others you can discover at *Whole Health Now*, whn.org.

Make sure to watch the movie, *Homeopathy, The Movie*, by Carol Boyce of Something to Say Productions. This will show you the impact homeopathy is having now around the world.

ASSIGNMENT #8

1. What is the meaning of *Genus epidemicus*?
2. What medicines were used for the Great Flu of 1918?
3. Who made homeopathy into a system of medicine? In what century?
4. Pick one homeopathic medicine and discuss its keynotes.

CHAPTER 9: BOTANICAL MEDICINE

Ah, the beauty of plants, medicinal plants full of goodness to strengthen our bodies and minds and then to be stirred, swallowed, or made into a tea or decoction to be used when a pathogenic virus is on the horizon.

Like homeopathy, botanical medicine is making a comeback in the general population in America, after both the damaging effects of the Rockefeller-Carnegie funded Flexner Report of 1910 and the obsession with antibiotics after World War II for every little sickness. This resurgence of interest and use of medicinal plants including in research is coming just in time and is a testimony to our deep connection with the earth and its many offerings and gives us comfort that we humans are not alone on this beautiful planet gone amok.

Thankfully, Traditional Chinese Medicine has thousands of years to back its validity in viral infections. Chinese and Taiwanese research has excellent research for "anti-influenza" plants and are snapping up kudos in COVID-19 although you never hear this from the mainstream media.

"I think it is the correct approach," says Cheng Yung-chi, a professor of pharmacology at Yale University School of Medicine. "The evidence is going to come, and we have to give it the benefit of the doubt."[1]

My interest in plants for a viral infection like influenza exploded when I heard about *Lomatium dissectum*, a root used traditionally for upper respiratory infections by the Washow people of Nevada when I went to Bastyr:

During the fall of 1918 when the influenza epidemic hit, Dr. E. Krebs Sr., M.D. of Carson City, NV (and the physician assigned by the US government to the Washoe) observed that the Washoe people were recovering. There was not a single death. Dr. Krebs made a crude preparation and tried it on non-Indians in San Francisco whom he said, "(They) just stopped dying." Dr. Krebs considered *Lomatium* specific in epidemic influenza and any accompanying pneumonia. His friend Max Barlow joined him in making it available.

Botanicals (herbs) and pharmaceuticals (drugs) each have their place on the healthcare spectrum, but drugs must be saved for serious situations. Plants, akin to homeopathy, are potent healers with minimal risk, produced at a very low cost that can be distributed widely. Even invasive plants considered noxious weeds are worthy of our curiosity and inspection. Banned in several states, they are seen as a threat to the local ecosystem and are eradicated posthaste, when they could be doing some good. Reading a book by herbalist Stephen Harrod Buhner, I first learned that invasive plants could appear where they are needed for diseases that are emerging in the area. One example is the Amur honeysuckle (*Lonicera maackii*), native to Asia and Russia but grows elsewhere including America. It has the reputation for crowding other plants and a weed killer like the extremely toxic glyphosate is used to eradicate it in Ohio (the Ohio Environmental Council brags about it) and elsewhere where it has not been banned. Honeysuckle, however, has the ability to reduce the number of eggs laid by the mosquito, *Aedes triseriatus*, a factor in several viral diseases including LaCrosse encephalitis that can result in seizures, paralysis and even coma. Apparently the more honeysuckle growing in an affected region, the less the incidence of this disease. And on top of the reduction of mosquitoes, the cause, honeysuckle contains anti-inflammatory compounds specific for reducing inflammation in the brain during an infection. Whoa, isn't that something to sit up and take notice of? I wonder if COVID-19 is spawning a plant that can detoxify glyphosate perhaps just by inhaling its aroma?

BOTANICAL RESEARCH

After over a century of being relegated to the bottom of the bin in medical treatment, seen as ignorant folklore, scientific inquiry is finally happening (if not enough) revealing that many plants, including so-called invasives, have bioactive plant compounds, so-called antiviral properties, second to none. I look forward to the time when children learn about plants in their urban or rustic environments as a matter of course, when they are able to go out and identify plants to help heal themselves and their communities.

Botanical researcher, Paul Bergner of the North American Institute of Medical Herbalism, emailed me, "The term 'antiviral' is imprecise. Unfortunately, the term implies all such herbs, or their constituents, somehow kill viruses directly, rather than enhancing host response." This is something to keep in mind as we discuss medicinals appropriate to an infectious disease.

Each strain of virus has its own unique presentation on its surface that allows it to scoot into its target host cell membrane (us). As discussed in chapter three, H (hemagglutinin) and N (neuraminidase) are the receptor sites in an influenza virus and although earlier thought the culprit was the ACE2 receptor for COVID-19 it is more likely receptor CD 147-cyclophilin. According to new research. (See chapter 7, COVID-19) This exact fitting, like a key to a lock, determines if a virus will infect us. Research from around the world is exposing the potential of plants as novel antiviral agents that inhibit formation of viral RNA or viral reproduction in a variety of ways. These bioactive plant compounds include polysaccharides, flavonoids, terpenoids, lignan, saponins, proteins, peptides...the list goes on and on.

Immunomodulating or adaptogenic effects on our cells by botanicals work through signaling pathways that alert various molecules, cells or receptors (like CD147 or H and N) to come together to shoo away a pathogenic virus. But it has been tricky to determine a plant's mode of healing on a human because much research begins in a Petri dish, making it difficult to determine the exact action of a plant on, or rather in, a human body.

One example is the mechanism of inhibition, how a plant interferes in the life cycle of the virus. This may be seen in a Petri dish, but it is difficult to correlate with a person swallowing a tincture or taking a capsule. Technology has not reached that stage.

It is worthwhile noting that although there has been talk that botanicals may be able to incite a cytokine storm, research in Traditional Chinese medicinal plants states the opposite.[2]

THE MAGIC OF POLYSACCHARIDES

So why do plants such as licorice or elderberry come up on our radar as showing they are helpful in a viral infection? The fact is we may not know exact mechanisms of action but we do know certain parts of a plant have what is termed an antiviral effect. Polysaccharides, isolated from different species of plants, are getting a lot of attention in scientific and botanical circles these days.

Polysaccharides come from plant cell walls and represent just one compound of many that are being referred to as biological response modifiers (BRMs) as part of the first line of defense as what enters the cell that will affect the nucleus thereby activating pathways and inducing production of pro-inflammatory cytokines such as TNF-alpha and IL-6, a huge benefit to pathogenic virus resistance, as long as a BRM remains in balance and doesn't end up as a cytokine storm.

Polysaccharides work through our macrophages,[3] the predominant white blood cell activated early on in a viral infection by TLRs (Toll-like receptors), complement receptors, and protein complexes like NF-kB. (Are you putting it all together with the immune system chapter and others?)

Additional plant mechanisms at work to increase our host resistance include TH-1/TH-2 balance, heat-shock proteins, and TLR (toll like receptors), and a host of other signaling pathways.[4]

TH-1/TH-2 BALANCE

TH stands for T-helper cells. Paul Bergner calls them the "quarterbacks" of the specific immune system. As someone who is not enamored by football, excluding Colin Kaepernick, I'd rather refer to T-helper cells as the brains, the motivator that amplifies both the cell-mediated (macrophages, T-killer cells) and the humoral (antibody) responses. These cells can remain undifferentiated or they can become either TH-1 or TH-2. TH-1 aligns with cell-mediated immunity and TH-2 with antibody production. This may create an imbalance, allowing one side to dominate. If this dominance is with TH-2 it can lead to viral overload due to a lack of cells to clear the antibodies tagged for the virus from the system. Events like this can happen in a chronic viral infection and/or due to repeated vaccinations, making it more difficult to recover. And it underscores the need for detoxification in any healing process.

AN EXAMPLE OF WHITE BLOOD CELL IMBALANCE

A possible case of antibody overload is now thought to occur with Echinacea spp. and autoimmune diseases as well as chronic fatigue syndrome and fibromyalgia. Echinacea increases white blood cells, including the lymphocytes, and if the system is already unbalanced with a predominance of TH-2 then the condition/disease could be aggravated. However, this is being disputed in scientific circles as I write. In any case, I'm giving Echinacea a pass here due to the possible role it plays in the rising incidence of autoimmune disease in general. (Echinacea has a soft spot in my heart being the first plant I studied at Bastyr and is high on my list as a blood cleanser.)

One of the reasons naturopathic physicians get such good results is that what causes TH-2 dominance includes immunizations, corticosteroids, depletion of glutathione and excess cortisol levels with corresponding DHEA deficiency that comes from stress. These are all conditions we either refrain from or balance daily in our clinics. And although plants can help regulate TH-2 dominance more research is needed.

HEAT-SHOCK PROTEINS

Heat-shock proteins are produced within the cell in response to stress. They augment the effectiveness of protein assembly and transport, thereby increasing immunity against cells infected with a virus.

Our body's defense mechanism may be activated by extremes of cold or hot (locally or systemically) that can work in the body's favor when a virus is on the prowl; hence the benefit of fever therapy, hydrotherapy and exercise[2] with a negative influence being an excess of refined sugar that decreases the effectiveness of the expression of heat-shock proteins, a reason to keep your blood sugar stable. (Licorice is helpful, as well as *Schisandra, Paenia,* Garlic and Turmeric.)[5]

MORE ON TOLL-LIKE RECEPTORS

Toll-like Receptors (TLR) are a recent discovery that elucidates previously unknown pathways. These don't come from the humoral and cell-mediated system—specific immunity of B and T-cell—but from macrophages and the complement system,[6] the non-specific side of our immune system. These defense cells detect chemicals that are specific to organisms like viruses, bacteria, etc., initiating a systemic response. Our old friends, the polysaccharides in plants, trigger this activity from the TLR, creating again an NSA situation, albeit in your body. Research is beginning to make specific connections.

RESEARCH GOING ON AROUND THE WORLD

Research groups around the world are investigating antiviral agents from native traditional plant medicine. (See the work of Jill Stansbury, ND.) These all either block viral entry, replication, assembly and release, or target virus-host-specific interactions.

Many North American plants have shown to be active against the influenza virus [3,6,7,8,9] we shall see in time in terms of COVID-19.[1,2,10] The list includes *Lomatium dissectum, Sambucus nigra* (elderberry) and *Glycyrrhiza glabra* (licorice), and it's looking good for *Osha* (chuchupate), *Rosa nutkana, Eleutherococcus senticosus* (roots), *Sanicula europaea, Bergenia ligulata, Nerium indicum, Holoptelea integrifolia,* even the cactus *Opuntia streptacantha.* (The latter has shown to act against an influenza virus according to research in British Columbia, Canada and reported all the way back in 1995![11] And then there is the freshwater algae, Spirulina, marine algae and other seaweeds with their array of metabolites—fucoidans, carrageenans, polyphenols and so on—we can use. (This is why I take phytoplankton daily.)

In China and Taiwan, clinical trials of plants are showing that Traditional Chinese Medicine (TCM) is a rich resource for novel antivirals including *Glycyrrhiza glabra, Chinese Bupleurum spp, Houttuynia, Isatis indigotica, Scropholia, Scutellaria,* flavonoids extracted from litchi seeds, herbacetin, epigallocatechin gallate

(EGG), and quercetin.[10]

85% of CoVID-19 patients in China have received Traditional Chinese Medicine (TCM). As of March 1, 2020, there are 303 ongoing clinical trials. Research continues in the United States and Taiwan.[1,10]

As for previously successful coronavirus plant antivirals for SARS 1 and MERS that might be active against COVID-19, we can add *Amelanchier alnifolia, Rosa nutken, Artemisia annua, Toona sinensis,* Rosemary (and other culinary herbs) and many more. [1,7]

One particular botanical presently being studied is *Sambucus Formosana Nakai* that has strong activity against human coronavirus NL63 (HCoVNL63).[12] Although similar to *Sambucus nigra* (elderberry) and can be helpful to fight a viral infection, it does not appear to inhibit COVID-19. The caffeic acid component[13] seems to be responsible in inhibiting replication and blocking attachment of the virus. Foods containing caffeic acid are in Clinical Nutrition.

Another botanical I am very excited about is Ashwagandha because it is an extraordinary adaptogenic plant (helps the body adapt to stress) that benefits the adrenals and thyroid, an all-around awesome plant that helps vitality and stamina that is so important before and after a severe viral infection. Research shows it can bind COVID-19.

BOTANICALS TO KNOW FOR INFLUENZA or COVID-19

Glycyrrhiza Glabra (Licorice)[1,3, 13,14,15]

Description: Small, pointy leaves and flower clusters.
Habitat/Family: Europe, Asia, North America, South America, and Australia.
Active Ingredient: Glycyrrhizin, the most frequently used Chinese herb contained in many TCM formulas,[6] is 50 times sweeter than sugar although may have an aftertaste some people don't like. Licorice candy is a misnomer since the taste comes from anise.
Function: This botanical has lots of great health benefits due to flavonoids, lignans, and other phytochemicals. Glycyrrhizin nudges the immune system to secrete more interferon, an antiviral chemical, and inhibits the virus from penetrating the cell to replicate

itself; much scientific evidence highlighting influenza and COVID-19 as noted; many trials show that it inhibits the viral cycle in vitro and also stimulates interferon-gamma production from t-cells, shown to inhibit replication of clinical isolates of SARS virus; antiviral against influenza, including H5N1 influenza a virus-infected cells; effective against SARS-associated coronavirus/ COVID-19; inhibits viral adsorption (creates a film on the surface) and penetration, soothes mucus membranes; has nine different natural expectorants to break up phlegm and ease coughing-shown it as effective as codeine; when deglycyrrhizinated, the active ingredient is removed to avoid hypertension because of potassium sparing.
History: From the latin term "*liquirtia*" that was based on the Greek term "*glukos riza*" or sweet root; used for centuries in China and rome for respiratory troubles and intestinal complaints.
Dosage: ¼ tsp solid extract three times a day or ½ to 1 tsp tincture a day; can double this or even triple for a brief period during a severe bout or pandemic.
Caution: Side effects may include high blood pressure, water retention, headache, lethargy, unbalanced potassium and sodium levels though unlikely during the short time of a viral infection; may be avoided by people with hypertension, kidney or liver problems or heart disease by substituting *Lomatium* or elderberry.

Lomatium dissectum[16]

Description: Root. First discovered by the Washoe tribe in Nevada.
Habitat/Family: Grows in the Pacific Northwest and northern Nevada; a rare species of the parsley family.
Active Ingredients: Chemically unique coumarins including pyranocoumarins and furanocoumarins
Function: It has a viro-static effect: it stops the growth of all viruses and is known to dramatically reduce viral counts; as a powerful antiviral and broad-spectrum plant antibiotic hence, it could constitute a great resource against COVID-19; it's my first choice in treating influenza; also beneficial when fighting pneumonia as well as chronic fatigue syndrome, HIV, sinusitis, bronchitis, and the common cold; it is currently being used in several clinics (most in Mexico) for clearing infection in cancer patients.
History: The Washoe called *Lomatium* "the dortza" meaning heap

powerful medicine. Dr. Krebs (see earlier) called it *Balsamea* because of its strong balsamic resins, and botanists named it *Leptotaenia dissecta* until 1942 when it was reclassified as *Lomatium dissectum*. Two other names include "biscuit-root" as the pulp was pounded into cakes, and "Indian carrot" due to its large taproot and that it is related to the common carrot; preparation by the Washoe: gathered in late autumn when the richest supply of volatile oil factions—containing the antiviral/antibiotic ingredient—are concentrated in the underground root, the Washoe cut up the root longitudinally, exposing the volatile oils that convert to a stable resin. They made a decoction by curing it in the sun before hanging it from the ceiling of their Hogan (home) to be used as needed. A pound of root is said to be a good amount to treat a case of fever for three days, the longest time needed to break a fever due to influenza or a pulmonary disease. Dr. Krebs worked with Max Barlow, an herbalist and writer (from *The Shepherd's Purse*) to formulate LDM-100, a *Lomatium dissectum* tincture.[14]

Dosage: Depends on the strength of the natural immune system; if the patient is very weak, start with just a few drops in water; this can be safely increased until it takes effect as ldm-100 is non-toxic.

Adults: 3 to 10 drops added to water or juice, 3 to 5 times a day, or more. Start low and work up over 7 days and then increase as needed.

Children: 3 to 4 drops in juice, 4 to 6 times daily.

Babies: 1 to 2 drops in water or juice.

Recovering alcoholics can add boiling water first and let it cool.

Caution: Do not use if pregnant or nursing.

Side Effects: A one-time detox rash may occur, hives that can be itchy and uncomfortable in up to 10% of patients using tincture…if so, change to powdered herbs in capsules; this reaction may be overcome quickly by taking dandelion root, Vitamin C and pantothenic acid to help the liver; fresh juices especially wheat grass also can help. Discontinue use if rash persists; it usually does not recur if administered again, say in a few weeks. The rash may surface due to an underlying chronic infection that is being cleared so although the rash is uncomfortable the end result can be a very happy consequence. May deplete friendly bacteria so take a higher dose of a probiotic. Since some species are poisonous it is best to order from a reputable company like Barlow Herbal.

Sambucus Canadensis Or Nigra (Black Elderberry)[17]

Description: A beautiful shrub, elderberry is a member of the honeysuckle family; the flowers, clustering in large numbers, turn into edible black or dark purplish berries rich in nutrition and healing substances like anthocyanins and flavonoids.

Habitat/Family: Found all over North America and Europe as well as Western Asia and North Africa in parks, woods and along riverbanks. Songbirds and small mammals love elderberries. White-tailed deer enjoy the twigs, foliage, and fruit. Nesting cover for small birds. In springtime its white flowers emit a particular scent, a bit sweet but rather repugnant as it has a bit of a rotting flesh smell since it attracts carrion flies to effect pollination.

Active Ingredient(s): Has high amounts of anthocyanin, a potent antioxidant; anthocyanins boost cytokines, the key messengers in the immune system; they also protect the mucous membranes including the sinuses and reduce swelling by decreasing inflammation; twice as much Vitamin C as an orange; high amount of Vitamin E; trace minerals; an even higher ORAC—oxygen radical absorbance capacity—than blueberry and cranberry; patented as the main ingredient of the drug, Sambucol, in Israel.

Function: Known to reduce symptoms of influenza by four days[18]; inhibits over ten strains of influenza virus in-vitro; immune-modulating activity stimulates production of certain cytokines leading to activation of phagocytes facilitating movement to inflamed tissues; increases cytokine (TNF) tumor-necrosis factor alpha by 5000% in healthy subjects along with inflammatory cytokines - IL-1, IL-6, IL-8, IL-10, TNF alpha[15]; prevents influenza virus from invading respiratory cells because of antivirin which helps neutralize the hemagglutinin spikes that allow the virus to enter the cell; some have compared it to the pharmaceutical zanamivir (Relenza) and other neuraminidase inhibitors; effective even for swine flu, H1N1.

History: Its genesis can be traced back to the Greek word "*sambuke*", meaning wind instrument; Native Americans/First Nation people used every part of the plant calling it the "tree of music"; long tradition like nettles as a "spring cure." They made tools like arrow shafts, pipes and flutes from the branches.

The word "elder" is from the Anglo-Saxon "aeld" meaning fire. The hollow stems of this plant were used to blow on flames to intensify the fire. An American sailor with arthritis accidentally discovered the health benefits of elderberry in 1899 by drinking wine infused with elderberries.

Dosage: Long term safety is unknown so treat for a maximum of 3 - 4 days; as a syrup extract: one tablespoon, four times a day; if standardized to 30-38%, 1-3 teaspoons three times a day; as a lozenge: several times a day; as a tea/decoction: two teaspoons of dried European elder flowers in a cup of hot water, steep, strain and drink several times a day; in powdered capsule form: 500mg 2- 3 times daily; liquid extract: 1:1.5 to 3 mls given 2- 3 times a day; tincture: 1:5: 1-5 mls 2- 3 times a day.

Caution: Elderberry may act as a diuretic and may increase the risk of dehydration; for diabetics, it may lower blood sugar levels making hypoglycemia a possibility; ask your oncologist if you're undergoing chemotherapy - it may interfere; don't combine with laxatives; for those with asthma and other respiratory conditions, don't use with Theophylline or only take reduce levels; avoid after organ transplants.

Side Effects: Has a small amount of cyanide producing glycosides that are released on digestion so to be consumed in small quantities raw to avoid nausea and vomiting; if if you are going to eat a lot, cook them.

Withania Somnifera (Ashwagandha) also known as Winter Cherry[19-25]

Description: A greyish, shrub with yellow or greenish flowers that are followed by small, spherical, orangish-red berries containing yellow, kidney-shaped seeds; cultivated widely as the whole plant for medicine, mostly the root and leaf, it grows three-to-five feet tall, mainly on waste land.

Habitat/Family[19]: Indigenous to Africa, northwestern states of India, also Pakistan, and Nepal and the Mediterranean.

Active Ingredient(s): The root and leaves have steroidal alkaloids and lactones known as withanolides which serve as hormone precursors that can convert into human physiologic hormones as necessary; they include withanolides for COVID-19 with the bulk of activity from Withaferin A for influenza as it acts against the neuraminidase in H1N1 and Withanolide D.

Function: The benefits of this plant are immense;[16,17,19-21] traditionally, it has been used as an aphrodisiac, liver tonic, anti-inflammatory agent, and astringent while more recently, to treat respiratory disorders such as bronchitis and asthma, ulcers, insomnia, and senile dementia; clinical trials indicate it has immunomodulatory properties and is anti-depressive for our purposes but there are many other therapeutic effects; it has an anxiolytic effect (anti-anxiety), it is an adaptogenic, shows promise as an antiviral, improves mitochondrial function; as a rejuvenative for men it increases vitality and "strengthens bone marrow, muscle and semen."[23] In the elderly it gives energy, in special need during COVID-19, decreases pain and inflammation and nervous debility; it benefits memory, and is also found useful in neurodegenerative diseases such as Parkinson's, Huntington's and Alzheimer's; additionally, it has GABA mimetic effect, shown to promote formation of dendrites.

History: The name comes from "ashwa" for horse and "gandha" for smell, and is meant to signify strength, although its second name means sedative. (This seeming incongruity becomes less confusing when you experience its benefits. Strength with calm is a close description to what one feels.) This is a much-revered plant known to help many conditions and as such has played a special role in Ayurvedic medicine for more than 3000 years.

Dosage: 500 mg a day or more (equal to 12 ml of tincture) ... doesn't seem to harm at higher doses. Caution with pregnancy and nursing, keep low.

Side Effects: Studies show very little risk; may interact with medications so if you are on thyroid, blood pressure or are diabetic; check with your integrated doctor for your particular case; if you have an allopathic doctor you may need them to do some research on this plant- it will be worth it.

Caution: Possible caution if on thyroid, blood pressure or diabetic meds; can be taken in pregnancy and while nursing but not in large amounts according to Deb Soule from Avena Botanicals writing in a newsletter of Maine Organic Farmers and Gardeners Association; there are reports of liver toxicity but this comes from impure plants.

Scutellaria[26,27]

(A possibility.) Various species. Can be useful for both Influenza and COVID-19. *S. lateriflora* has been used in the West for weakness after influenza; *S. baicalensis* is a Chinese plant that is being studied for its influence to inhibit the influenza virus in vivo (mice)-isolate baicalin (inhibitor) and SARS and is being presently studied for COVID-19; Baicalin is an isolate that was first studied by Frank Rosetti and Judy Mikovits in the 1990s; a star in TCM (Traditional Chinese Medicine), it acts by inhibition of cathepsin L, a lysosomal cysteine protease, an enzyme active in the antigen (*i.e.* virus) processing through protein degradation; another isolate, wogonin, a flavonoid, is also being evaluated presently-it shows an up-regulation of interferon (IFN)-induced antiviral signaling. See Resources for Baicalin powder (1/2 tsp twice a day) from bioPURE™.

ADDITIONAL PLANTS FOR SPECIFIC USE:

Expectorants: These support the flow of mucous. (see Part Four)

- Licorice - *Glycyrrhiza glabra*
- Coltsfoot - *Tussilago farfara*
- Cottonwood – *Populus fremontii*
- Fennel - *Fructus foeniculi*
- Gumweed - *Grindelia camporum*
- Anise - *Fructus anisi*
- Hyssop - *Hyssopus officinalis*
- Elecampane - *Inula helenium*
- White horehound - *Marrubium vulgare*
- Wild cherry - *Prunus serotina*
- Yerba santa* - *Eriodictyon californicum*

- *This "Sacred Herb" is California's preeminent medical plant...indigenous Californians have use this for centuries for all respiratory conditions, loosens chest mucus.

Any plants with berberine, curcumin and hesperidin can increase mucin release by directly acting on airway mucin-secreting cells; water is a great expectorant as well; lemon for alkalinity and cleansing can be added.

Demulcents: These increase mucus; you do not want dry mucous membranes as these are vital as a barrier to the outside, guarding against pathogens and environmental irritants.

- *Malva* (mallow)
- *Althea rosea* (hollyhock)
- Prickly Pear Cactus (opuntia, nopal)

Decongestants: Decrease swelling of mucous membranes; lessen the blockage.

- Elderflower......contains quercetin, a natural antihistamine-steam over a kettle (careful) or take a hot shower (followed by room temperature so your energy isn't depleted)

Antitussive: Good for a spasmodic cough that is keeping you up. Hedera Helix (Ivy Leaf) Cough syrup.

Diaphoretics: These induce perspiration to cool a fever: works by shifting blood to the capillaries of the skin; heat escapes, thus speeding the elimination of toxins.

- Lobelia - Lobelia inflata - great respiratory herb used with steam (taught to herbalist, Samuel Thomson (1769-1843) by the First Nations/Native Americans.)

- Elderberry - Sambucus nigra - as above
- Peppermint - Mentha piperita - helps with headaches
- Holy Basil - Ocimum sanctum – relaxation
- Lemon Balm - Melissa officianalis antiviral, relaxing (don't

take if you have hypothyroidism)

- Oregano - Origanum vulgare (use the concentrated essential oil for best results)
- Osha – Chuchupate - for pneumonia but seek professional help if get to that stage
- Saffron - Crocus sativus - great antioxidant

Adaptogens: These are plants that have a nonspecific response, boosting the body's ability to resist multiple stresses; they can normalize an immune system response that is overstimulating, possibly on its way to a cytokine storm. Choose from:

- Ashwagandha
- *Rhodiola rosea* (Arctic root)
- *Tulsi* (Holy Basil)
- *Ganoderma lucidum* (Reishi mushroom)[11]: fabulous preventive to build general immunity and for chronic viral load (helps balance TH-2) but no research has found it active against influenza virus; unknown about COVID-19 at this time; alcohol preparations do not contain plant polysaccharides so probably useless; get fresh or dried mushrooms; increases systemic immunity by its polysaccharide content increasing cytokines from monocytes, macrophages and lymphocytes and through their action on TLRs; homeopathically speaking, this plant is being investigated by German homeopath Anna Schade who calls this a medicine for our times.
- *Eleutherococcus senticosus* (Siberian ginseng)[30]: it enhances cell-mediated immunity (TH-1) and through toll-like receptors. According to Paul Bergner most products in the US and Canada are useless; only HerbPharm® of Williams, Oregon, markets a product made according to Russian (the original research) specifications, concentrated to 2:1 strength; noticeable activity should result in 1 to 2 days; it can result in anxiety and insomnia.
- Birch: Use of these leaves off hot and moist rocks to cleanse the lung…to help expel toxins; Russians are known to use switches of green birch twigs aka Birch Broom to thrash the

body

- *Tylophora*: an Ayurvedic medicinal plant, known since 1891 to help respiratory disorders; Its active ingredients, alkaloids, include tylophorin.

MORE TCM RESEARCH

- *Angelica sinensis* (Dang Gui) and *Salvia miltiorrhiza*[30] (Danshen) have shown to inhibit the inflammatory cytokine High Mobility Group Box 1 protein (HMGB1) in mice[5]; also cited was *Trifolium pretense* (red clover), a possible influenza treatment due to its anti-inflammatory properties.
- Another study evaluated anti-neuraminidase activity in five traditional Chinese herbs - *Duchesnea indica, Liquidambar formosana, Lithospermum erythrorhizon, Melia toosendan* and *Prunella vulgaris*; all exhibited strong inhibitory activities to NA and antiviral effects against influenza A virus; *Melia toosendan* significantly reduced the death rate and prolonged survival in H1N1 infected mice;[5,7] a mouse study discusses the effects of ginseng[10] and salvia on early immune responses during influenza virus infection. Ginseng induced high levels of cytokines IL-4 and Il- 5 in cells while Salviae increased IFN-y and IL-2 cytokines producing splenocytes; both act as mucosal adjuvants against influenza virus as well as immune modulators, at least in mice.

LASTLY, a mention...

Over 300 clinical trials of TCM plants are being studied in China and Taiwan, including ancient herbal extract formulas,[2,3,10] as treatments for upper respiratory infections.

- *Yin Qiao San Fructus Forsythiae, Flos Lonicerae, Radix Platycodonis, Herba Menthae, Herba Lophatheri, Radix Glycyrrhizae, Herba Schizonepetae,* Fermented soybean, *Fructus arctii,* and *Rhizoma Phragmitis;* an antiviral, anti-inflammatory and immune regulator.
- *Yu Ping Feng San Astragali radix, Astragalus membranaceus, Atractylodes macrocephala,* and *Saposhnikoviae Radix.*
- It seems these formulas can modulate T cells to enhance host response with one study showing that in the control group

.4% were infected with zero of those infected who received this formula; these will be evaluated at a later date.

As you can see there are sooooooo many plants that are being studied (although not enough considering how much we need them and how many there are on the planet) that may possibly be helpful in treating a viral airborne infection. So why oh why aren't we giving these to immunocompromised folks right now???

DOSAGES

This is the tricky part as there are so many variants in terms of the metabolism of our body and the botanical preparation itself. Individual differences in constitution, particular sensitivities, varying degrees of absorption and so on influence how much is needed.

There are many ways a botanical medicine can be served up – tea, a stronger infusion, a decoction, tincture, loose powder, dried in a capsule, or made into a tablet. And you can learn to make them all if you choose but if you are new to this buying store bought preparations that are standardized (have a certain amount of active ingredient in a certain amount of the medicinal plant) from a reputable botanical company (see Resources) may be the best way to go until you gain more and experience. The suggested dose will be on the label. But remember, this is a suggestion and is based on a 150 lb. body. Add or subtract from there.

When you are making your own you will need to experiment with the dose, carefully. Start with a very small dose and work up (called titrating) if you aren't getting the results you were hoping for.

If this seems too complex or worrisome, simply offer teas, use hydrotherapy and find out the *genus epidemicus*.

Clark's Rule for children: Child's weight in lbs (pounds) divided by 150, then multiply by adult dose.

LATIN TERMS*

q.d.	once a day
b.i.d.	twice a day
t.i.d.	three times a day
q.i.d.	four times a day
ic	between meals
ac	before meals
Pc	after meals
W	With
aq cal	hot water
aq ge	cold water
Gtt	Drops
prn	taken as needed
m	Morning
n	Night
Ca	About

- *Books to consult are in Resources.

ASSIGNMENT #9

1. What are the main botanicals to consider in influenza?
2. What are two you could use for COVID-19 and why?
3. Pick one plant of the main four listed and discuss.
4. How many ways can you think of to use a plant to heal?

CHAPTER 10: HYDROTHERAPY INCLUDING ESSENTIAL OILS

The next "Ahh, the bliss" is for water, hydrotherapy, seemingly magical in how it helps to heal. Its ability to decrease pain, help one relax and detoxify are all reasons for utilizing this easily accessible non-toxic, and yes, most of the time, delightful, treatment. (A cold shower after warm or hot is delightful afterward. ☺)

Animals understand this: they are known to bathe an injured limb in a flowing stream. Cold, hot, fast or slow moving, it increases or decreases our circulation to bring needed nutrients to our cells and tissues and takes away waste to ensure elimination of toxic by-products of metabolism or environmental contaminants from food, drugs, and pollution.[1] There it augments autophagy, our inherent detoxifier of any detritus from damaged cells or viruses.

Taking saunas has been reported to decrease the number of colds in one study. In addition, it has been implicated in improvement of almost of every health issue every time it was studied.[1-3]

I first experienced intentional water treatment at Bastyr University when it was called John Bastyr College of Naturopathic Medicine. I learned to follow a warm or hot shower with cold to boost the immune system and feel more energetic, invigorated. And then there were the wet sheet treatments along with the cold socks treatments I endured from classmates in order to pass Constitutional Hydrotherapy class. Not easy but the effects, as blood is manipulated and healing is generated, make it worth it, if you are ill or rundown.

Hydrotherapy has a long and regal as well as common history. Ancient Egyptian royalty were known to use water medicinally by soaking in large warm pools mixed with oils and flowers. And it may have been even earlier in Asia—China, Japan, Tibet and India—where natural hot springs, rich in minerals, were used to not only cleanse but heal the body, dispelling toxins and encouraging blood flow to increase oxygenation. And we probably all know about Russian and Korean spas, Japanese baths, even if we haven't experienced them.

I was excited to discover a spa in Tibet in the middle of nowhere or everywhere, depending on your view…One thing's for sure, water heals, and most cultures use it…instead of pills at times. Can you imagine?

Travelling to India, Ecuador, Vanuatu, China, I realized almost all countries have their favorite hydrotherapy treatment whether through hot rocks, swirling waters, steam or just a dunk in the ocean. In Los Angeles, where I presently live, I go to Beverly Hot Springs, a Korean spa with real hot springs, the only one in the city. (Here is their blurb (abbreviated): "The spa is fed by a strong flow of 96 to 105 degree water from the artesian well that Richard S. Grant found when he bought the land–then a wheat field–to subdivide for a housing development in 1910. Dug near the turn of the century by drillers looking for oil, the 2,200-foot well supplied water to early residents of the area near Western Avenue and Beverly Boulevard until city water mains were installed in 1915. Later the water was sold as drinking water bottled as "Wonder Water" under the Angelus Club label with the slogan "Nature's Own Formula." The water was especially popular among red-eyed men who found the sodium bicarbonate and other minerals it contains soothing on Monday mornings. According to a chemical analysis made in 1931, the alkaline water contains sodium bicarbonate, (the major mineral at 82.6 grains per gallon), silica, iron and aluminum oxides, magnesium carbonate, sodium carbonate, sodium sulfate and sodium chloride." Too bad there's only the one in L.A., and not every mile!)

Steam, as First Nations/Native Americans demonstrated to Samuel Thomson, the founder of a botanical medical system, can be inhaled with plants like lobelia, menthol or eucalyptus, all helpful for lung tissue as well as bronchial airways. These can alleviate constriction, allowing mucus and other fluids to be dispelled from the lungs and therefore increasing oxygen. This also acts as a detox since the detritus of spent organisms (virus and bacteria) that have been killed by the white blood cells are removed through mucus and other fluids.

METHOD OF ACTION

How hydrotherapy works is that water can change temperature

and pressure in the body. These changes are sensed by nerve endings in the skin and muscles and results in neural "reflex effects" that are controlled by the brain and spinal cord. The most important of these are vasodilation and vasoconstriction that respectively relax or tense the blood vessels. This physical change causes changes in the rate of blood flow and then any metabolic functions related to blood flow. This can happen systemically (whole body) or locally (in one area of the body).

Hot and cold water act in different ways. Cold water and ice cause the body to try to conserve heat. Blood vessels constrict, decreasing the amount of blood that flows through them. Blood flow then is diverted from the extremities (less essential) to the core of the body and its organs (more essential to the body as a whole). The pores of the skin close, sweat glands shut down, muscles tense yet certain organs like the adrenal glands become more active. This can be useful for short periods of time.

Heat increases blood flow through blood vessels, increasing blood flow to the extremities and skin as well as relaxing muscles. Many ailments of a viral infection will be helped with water due to this change in blood flow with the ability to clean the system of inflammatory debris. Hydrotherapy protocols are designed to ensure various combinations of water temperature, water pressure and points of delivery. For example, by increasing the rate of blood flow in the body (heating it up) your white blood cells[3]—the worker bees of the immune system—work faster and more efficiently. This can also release endorphins, the body's pain killers as well as helping the body to heal. If you do an alternating hot and cold series, they will act in the same way but by a pumping action.

PRECAUTIONS: Be careful not to go to extremes of hot or cold, especially if you or the person is weak. If in doubt talk to your integrated doctor (iPCP), not everyone is suitable...milder treatments may be advisable.

CONSTITUTIONAL HYDROTHERAPY

Sitz baths, saunas, showers, poultices, wraps, inhalations and colon irrigation all fall under this category. There is evidence that the delivery of minerals or herbs adds to the benefit from the thermal and mechanical effects of water.[1] Hydrotherapy gives you several ways to manipulate the positive effects on the bloodstream that will transport nourishment to cells, specifically those in the endocrine system or neural pathways that are so important in healing the whole body.

The primary goal of constitutional hydrotherapy is to increase core body temperature. It can also lower blood pressure, reduce pain, lower elevated liver enzymes (so common these days) and for our purposes to increase white blood cells. One treatment may be all that is necessary although a series is most likely needed. This is something that can be done as soon as anyone mentions "epidemic."

TERMS

- COMPRESS: A compress is a soft cloth or pad of some type that can provide moisture, either hot or cold. Herbs, in any form including aromatherapy may be added as needed.
- POULTICE: Poultices are thick, usually water-based, hot glops that contain herbs, minerals, oils, etc. that can be spread on the chest (or other area) directly.
- TOWEL WRAPS: These are strips of cloth soaked in hot or cold water that can be wrapped around a body part, afterwards covered with a dry towel, and then left to dry.
- INHALATIONS: Inhalations allow hot or cold water to be delivered into the lungs through the nose; they usually carry some medicinal herb to enhance lung health.

AMPLIFY YOUR DAILY ROUTINES

- Make sure to keep hydrated at all times but especially when you are ill.
- Increase lymphatic flow by drinking alkaline water.
- Rule of thumb is to drink half your body weight in ounces per day, *i.e.* 140 lbs then 70 ounces.
- Showers: A simple hot and cold alternating shower can work wonders not just to boost the circulation and immune system but as a refreshing way to calm the mind. Go back and forth

three times between hot and cold (or warm and cool if you are feeling weak). The idea is to alternate hot/cold…hot/cold...hot/cold - 90 seconds hot, 30 seconds cold or 30 seconds hot and 10 seconds cold. Always finish with cold and make sure to dry thoroughly.

- Bath or Footbath: Make sure to drink water before and afterwards, filter the water by Bath Ball and add:
  1 cup baking soda
  2 cups Epsom salts
  2 cups Dead Sea Salt (optional)
  Water shouldn't be too hot. Make sure to dry thoroughly.
  Soak at least twenty minutes.
- During sickness: may augment with a diaphoretic or sweat-inducing herb like elderberry flowers or other suggestions in the Botanical chapter.

COLON IRRIGATION/COLONICS

This is like a high-tech enema without the high tech…I have found so many professionals including many naturopathic physicians who don't understand how helpful colonics can be. They will not deplete your bacterial flora but will help immensely to boost your immune system by detoxifying your body.

- Do one as soon as you hear the word epidemic.
- In fact, do three, a day or two apart.
- Once you're ill you can try using a colema board over your toilet (or another DIY method).
- Just be careful.

THUMPING THE THYMUS

Your thymus gland is located just below the hollow of your clavicles in the center of your upper chest. It stimulates white blood cell production and so helps to boost your immunity.

- Using the side of a fist (or tips of your fingers if you are feeling fragile) …
- Lightly thump your thymus for 30 to 40 seconds.

LYMPHATIC BRUSHING

- With a natural bristle brush on dry skin draw circular motions upward from your feet to torso and from fingers to chest.
- Always work towards the heart, the direction the lymph flows.
- This will make sure it is moving forward, getting rid of toxins.

MASSAGE

Massage is not only a great way to relax but it gets the lymph moving, toxins eliminated. There are many types: even a foot massage on your own feet if necessary, can be extremely helpful.

NASAL SPRAY

Works wonders in prevention especially.

- Purpose: To clear the nose of any virus or bacteria, and/or mucus.
- Preparation: Have it handy in a dry container. Use one teaspoon baking soda with three teaspoons salt (no additives).
- Spray bottle (emptied): Add one teaspoon to one cup of distilled, filtered or water that has been boiled and cooled.
- Spray once or twice in each nostril four times a day.

NASAL LAVAGE

- Use a Neti Pot or a bulb syringe with lukewarm water and 1 tsp. sea salt or Himalayan salt to 2 cups of water.
- Over a sink tilt your head forward so that you are looking down into the sink. Insert the spout into one nostril, let's say the right. Keep breathing through your mouth. Turn your head to the right and let water move into the right nostril and exit the left nostril.

- The goal is to feel the water pass through your sinuses; some may come out through your mouth… no problem… just spit it out.
- Repeat for the left nostril.
- To end, blow out any remaining water through both nostrils 10 to 15 times over the sink. Don't block one nostril as that may affect the eustachian tube in your ear.

MUSTARD PACK

Mustard seed has been used for thousands of years for respiratory illness. This is a recipe that can be applied to the chest to increase circulation, stimulate the immune system, and alleviate lung conditions. It attracts blood, draws out toxins and helps bring up and clear congestion. It is safe and inexpensive.

MUSTARD PACK			
Supplies	1 cup organic flour (consider sprouted and gluten free, I'm serious) 1 Tbsp mustard	Directions	1. Make a paste 2. Apply to the chest or back over the protective smear of coconut oil. 3. Cover with a hot wet towel and leave on for twenty minutes, checking often. 4. Finish with an icy cold washcloth or small towel. 5. Make sure to keep warm.

CAUTION:

- The area can be red for hours, this is normal.
- Can be done once to three times a day and can be repeated on the back to get more direct access to the lungs.
- Be careful not to burn the skin - check often every few minutes especially with children or elders who are weak and having difficulty communicating.
- You can rub coconut oil over the area first to prevent burning and/or blistering.

WARMING SOCKS

This is particularly effective for fever and nasal congestion. Usually done before going to bed to help induce sleep but can be done at any time.

WARMING SOCKS			
Supplies	One pair cotton socks and one pair wool socks, preferably 100% cotton and at least 90% real wool.	Directions	1. Soak the foot part of the cotton socks in an ice bucket or cold tap water (depending on strength of the patient: the weaker the patient = the milder the temperature) and wring them out thoroughly. 2. If your feet are cold, soak them in a basin of hot water (or bathtub) for a few minutes until they are hot and pink. 3. Take your feet out of the water and quickly dry them off. Immediately put on the cold wet cotton socks and then put the wool socks on. 4. Lie down in bed, keeping the feet covered all night. 5. You should fall asleep after the initial shock which is why it's a great technique to do just before going to bed. 6. Your feet should warm up in a few minutes and congestion will usually begin to be relieved within 30 minutes. 7. It will often work better than a decongestant or antihistamine to relieve congestion during sleep. 8. It usually takes 4 hours for the socks to dry completely. 9. The feet will be warm, and symptoms will be improved if not gone. 10. Can be repeated during the night (no need to warm the feet in water in this case as they will be warm now) or on consecutive nights.

WET SHEET TREATMENT

WET SHEET TREATMENT			
Supplies	Cotton sheet, bucket of ice water, wool blanket; along the same line as the above Warming Socks this is done with sheets. We will call you B, and your helper A.	Directions	1. A soaks a cotton sheet in a bucket of ice water and squeezes out as much water as possible before spreading it over the bed onto a thick blanket. (Put something under the blanket to save the mattress) 2. B lies down on the wet sheet quickly and A wraps the sheet like a mummy tightly around B, leaving B's head out only. 3. The wool blankets are then wrapped around A.

Use blank areas on pages to record your notes!

ALTERNATING HOT and COLD SINUS COMPRESS

To clear the sinuses.

ALTERNATING HOT & COLD SINUS COMPRESS			
Supplies	Two face cloths, hot water and cold water.	Directions	1. Soak one cloth in hot water and wring out so it's damp but not dripping. 2. Place over nose and eyes and sinuses and leave it on for 3 minutes. 3. The second cloth is soaking in cold water (not ice cold). 4. Wring out and place over hot cloth and flip, removing the hot cloth and leaving the cold one. 5. Leave for 30 seconds. 6. Repeat this alternating sequence two more times for a total of three alternating sequences of three minutes hot and 30 seconds cold. You can do the nasal lavage after this for a deeper clearing.

NASAL LUBRICATION

This Ayurvedic treatment acts as a barrier between nasal passages and an unwanted virus. (Also good for people with sleep apnea and perhaps Alzheimer's because the oil can leak into the brain, a good thing apparently, and may be why Indians have a lower incidence of Alzheimer's.)

NASAL LUBRICATION			
Supplies	Dropper bottle organic sesame oil	Directions	1. Fill a dropper bottle with organic sesame oil. 2. Tip your head back and drop one drop in each nostril. 3. Or you can drop some oil into your palm and using your little finger apply the oil to the inside of your nostrils. (MAKE SURE TO WASH YOUR HANDS first if doing the second way.) 4. Inhale deeply a few times, allowing the oil to fall into your sinus cavities. Don't worry if some drips down your throat. 5. Wipe away excess oil.

You can do this morning and night especially if you live in a polluted city like Los Angeles where there are all sorts of particulates in the air that can irritate the nasal passages.

FEVER THERAPY

Naturopathic physicians do not see fever as the enemy but rather something that is essential to healing a viral infection. Fever is one of the body's best defenses. Often, however, fever doesn't happen, especially in the beginning, and we need to induce an artificial one. Do not do this if you have a fever or are suffering a chronic illness without consulting your healthcare provider.

FEVER THERAPY			
Supplies	Oral thermometer, very hot bath; before bed or make sure to have a few hours; lots of alkaline water...drink before, during and after.	Directions	1. Get into the bath and add water as hot as you can. (Obviously be careful especially with children.) 2. Take your temperature with the thermometer regularly while in the bath. After your temperature reaches 101 degrees F stay in the bath an additional 20 minutes. 3. This is the goal: 20 minutes. You will hopefully break into a heavy sweat. 4. Drink tepid, not cold water, as much as you can. 5. After 20 minutes get out of the bath carefully (you might feel faint) so don't stand up too quickly. 6. Dry off quickly, cover your head with a towel and put on absorbent clothing like heavy cotton pajamas or robe with socks. 7. Quickly get into bed before you cool down-you will feel hot, uncomfortably so, and will be sweating profusely. 8. Remain covered. 9. After 45 minutes to two hours you should be cooled off. 10. Remove wet clothing making sure not to be chilled. Follow with Wet Sock Treatment if planning to stay in bed.

ESSENTIAL OILS/AROMATHERAPY

Although this should technically be in the Botanical section this goes nicely with hydrotherapy as things you can do on your own. Homeopathy isn't easy and you may want to take an antiviral botanical on the advice of an expert, but this chapter allows for experimentation while being safe.

Cathey Clack Painter is a traditional naturopath and essential oils educator. I met Cathey while working on this book and discussed my desire for having essential oils listed as options for immune health. This is a compilation of her and my recommendations. For more information about essential oils, you can visit her website, catheypainter.com. She stresses, "It is always very very important to stress quality when it comes to using essential oils. In the U.S. you can call your oil 100% pure if it has just 1 drop of pure essential oil, the rest could be olive oil, etc. I recommend doTerra® essential oil, I had used another brand and never got results."

Just make sure the essentials are of the highest quality, like anything you buy for your health. This is so important. Lead and other toxins can be found in lower quality products. Don't take the chance!

APPLICATION

The fabulously seductive smells of essential oils stimulate or soothe our olfactory system while cleansing, sedating and killing germs. Like arnica in homeopathy, lavender will sell you on aromatherapy. You can use single oils or combine oils.

Preparation (several different ways):

- Apply directly to palms or soles of the feet. Rub in.
- Add carrier oil to a glass container, shake vigorously to blend. Inhale.
- Add water to a spray bottle, add essential oil and shake…then spritz.
- Add to a diffuser or aroma lamp.
- Carrier oils must be organic and of top quality: hemp oil,

olive oil, coconut oil (FCO), avocado oil, jojoba oil, grapeseed oil. (Never skimp on quality- it's not worth your health.)

- (FCO=fractionated coconut oil meaning lauric acid and other long chain fatty acids have been removed so the oil stays liquid at lower temperatures and is more easily absorbed by the skin.)

CLEANING THE SICK ROOM (using non-harmful substances)

Take a 32 oz glass spray bottle, add 2/3 water, 1/3 vinegar. I personally use a Protective Blend from doTERRA® called On Guard which has been proven to kill 99.99% of all microbes...viruses and bacteria. Just add 10 drops to your spray bottle...and use on doorknobs, and countertops. OnGuard® contains the following essential oils: Wild Orange, Clove, Cinnamon, Eucalyptus and Rosemary.

- **Aromatically:** One of the fastest ways to get benefits from essential oils is to breathe them in...either directly from the bottle, or add a drop to your palms, rub hands together and cup mouth and nose and take 10 deep breaths, or diffuse. Another benefit of using oils aromatically is they are directly linked to the amygdala, which is the part of our brain that processes emotions. The amygdala responds to smells. Improving emotions is very important for a strong immune system.
- **With a Diffuser:** Place a small bowl of water with 5 to 8 drops of essential oil with a tea candle (beeswax or soy, not paraffin). The heat from the candle allows the essential oil to diffuse into the air, making its way to your nose and lungs. These can kill germs as well as moisten the respiratory tract.

OILS FOR YOUR BODY

- **Topically:** Apply oils to the bottom of your feet, which is very porous. Within minutes the body uptakes the oil and every cell in your body is surrounded by molecules from the oil. You can also apply topically to the skin as needed. If the oil is hot or spicy, it is best to dilute it with FCO, the rule of thumb is for 1 teaspoon of FCO add 1 or 2 drops of oil.

- **Dosage:** Five drops of the essential oil in a carrier oil, up to five times a day for adults, is a good place to start. Halve this for children, so 2- 3 drops and babies starting with one drop.

ANTIVIRALS FOR PREVENTION AND IN THE SICK ROOM[5,6,7]

Essential oils shown with significant anti-influenza virus properties:

Melissa essential oil (lemon balm) - probably the most powerful antiviral essential oil. (Painter's favorite) *Not for use for people with hypothroidism.

- You can apply topically…best to dilute it with carrier oil such as fractionated coconut oil (FCO)
- You can also take 1 drop to 2 oz of water internally for prevention.
- OR 1 drop 4x a day internally when suffering from a virus.

Thyme essential oil - use for colds, flus & viruses, in capsules or inhale.

- Caution against high use during pregnancy or for those with epilepsy or high blood pressure.
- NOTE: Red thyme and white thyme come from the same plant. Red Thyme oil is a first distillation and very strong. Be careful with the elderly and children. But in a super influenza this is what you want to use, although white thyme oil can be substituted. It is simply more dilute being the second distillation and less potent. It is better for everyday uses. See Recipes for making an easy and powerful concoction from thyme.

MORE ANTI INFLUENZA VIRALS:

- *Citrus bergamia* (Bergamot oil)
- *Lavandula officinalis* (Lavender oil)
- *Eucalyptus globulus* (Eucalyptus oil)
- *Cinnamomum zeylanicum* (Cinnamon leaf oil)
- *Pinus sylvestris* (Pine oil)
- *Melaleuca viridiflora* (Tea tree oil)
- *Cymbopogon flexuosus* (Lemongrass oil)
- *Pelargon graveleons* (Geranium oil)
- Marjoram, Clary Sage and Anise were shown to have some but not a lot of activity against the influenza A virus.
- Oregano essential oil - known as nature's most powerful antibiotic.
    - use with extreme caution, it is extremely hot and spicy.
    - to take internally you must put in a capsule and top off with FCO.
    - apply diluted with FCO to the bottom of your feet at night as you crawl into bed.
    - If you're suffering from a virus, take 2-3 drops in a capsule 3-4 times a day and apply to the bottom of your feet for 7 days, then stop the protocol.
    - Some experts believe oregano oil is hard on the liver. Dr. Cass Ingram, (*101 Uses for Wild Oregano Oil*) the world's #1 expert on Oregano Oil, says it is not damaging to the liver if it is pure Oregano Oil.
- Yarrow - helps with allergies.
    - Take internally in a capsule and apply to the bottom of the feet and down spine.
- Black Pepper essential oil - while not antiviral, it helps promote respiratory and lymphatic drainage and cleansing.
    - Best to take internally in a capsule.
    - Add 1 drop to your morning coffee; keep in mind that coffee is a delivery system to the nervous system.

SPECIFIC FOR THE SICK ROOM

For inhalation or by careful application to the patient's skin with a few drops mixed in carrier oil, coconut preferred.

DISINFECTANTS (FOR THE ROOM):

- Lavender, rosemary, pine, tea tree and sage

FEVER REDUCER:

- Peppermint, chamomile, or lemon as a cool compress to the head or add to aroma diffuser.

ACHY JOINTS AND SORE MUSCLES:

- Add up to six drops to a carrier oil with ginger, rosemary, and/ or lavender.
- Massage into the area.

CONGESTION/MUCUS:

- Cedarwood, peppermint and/ or rosemary
- You can massage these oils into the chest with carrier oil or use an aroma lamp.
- Or you can tilt your head over hot water that has a few drops of the essential oil. Breathe in deeply.

GARGLES:

- For gargles, place one or two drops on a teaspoon of salt, dissolve in warm salty water; you can temper with tea tree, lemon, sage or thyme, garlic and ginger.

ESSENTIAL OILS IN RECOVERY

- Add to bath salts: lavender, ylang ylang, thyme, rosemary, basil, or lemon.

ASSIGNMENT #10

1. How does hydrotherapy heal?
2. Discuss one technique in depth *i.e.* wet sock treatment.
3. Name two essential oils you can try in a viral infection and why.
4. Name the ingredients of an essential oil formula to use instead of a toxic substance to wash your hands and clean counters?

CHAPTER 11: CLINICAL NUTRITION

A poor diet squanders a healthy immune system. Exactly what you don't want when you are fighting off a virus, of any type. Good clean food (organic if possible, therefore less chance of toxins) boosts your immune system through your gut, allowing your lymph system to get the wastes out so vitamins and minerals are maximally absorbed, increasing the oxygenation of tissue and the body's ability to repel unwanted pathogens. As well, your gut must be able to break down protein into amino acids easily.

The best dietary plan must be considered long before a virus is on the horizon. Junk food (bad fats, sugar, food additives) will lower your body's virus-fighting capabilities so if this is a big part of your diet please re-think this immune-strangling habit, at least until after the super virus has run its course.[1] Learning to love fresh vegetables and fruit isn't that difficult! Remember your taste buds have taken a hit with the sugar[2] and bad fats and fake tastes; they and your body will be thrilled when you take control. Avoid processed sugar and artificial sweeteners at all costs! These have been shown to make our immune system useless against pathogens.[3] This is especially important for people with underlying disorders such as diabetes.[4]

The easiest way to change food habits is to start going to a farmer's market weekly and checking out the colors and textures of fresh vegetables and fruits before tasting one or five. Make an effort to choose even one a week to become acquainted with.

For those of you who believe your diet needs no changes try to be open that it might need some tweaking. There are a number of reasons for this. One is the concept of clean food, food grown without chemicals. So, no matter what your food choice—vegan, vegetarian, Mediterranean, paleo, etc.—make sure to choose organic anything. Toxic residues from pesticides along with antibiotics have the ability to displace the minerals our body needs to function optimally. The other side of this is that a depletion of minerals in the soil is catastrophic to our health and may be the number one reason we as a species continue to rack up medical bills due to various types of sickness. Without a full quota of micronutrients [5] like adequate protein, minerals, and vitamins our bodies can't guarantee a healthy immune system, leaving us open to a virus or bacteria or fungi.

One major fact to consider is that our gut or gastrointestinal tract is an open tube (to what comes in from the outside and what goes back out) and therefore it must have a way to defend itself against harmful substances. In recent years we have learned that our gut harbors over two-thirds of our immune system. This is like having a second brain and corresponding nervous system ready to do the job necessary to keep our digestion flowing instead of waiting to engage the brain. This is especially helpful when we are sick or unconscious.

A HEALTHY LYMPH AND GUT

Good clean food generates a healthy lymph system, the garbage disposal system of the body. This waste system is essential to maintain wellness and prevent disease. Avoid constipation. This cannot be overemphasized. Otherwise the gut will breed unwanted bacteria, becoming a stockpile of toxins that interfere with the immune system. Probiotics, digestive enzymes including proteolytic enzymes ensure beneficial flora, keep your digestion running smoothly, helping to break down food and making sure it is absorbed properly. Fiber, as an anti-constipating agent and lectins from legumes have been shown to be potent anti-microbials and immune regulators.[5,6] Therefore, it is imperative to consume properly cooked (see legume recipes) beans and lentils to prevent infections.

FERMENTED FOODS MEANS INCREASED BENEFICIAL GUT BACTERIA

Beneficial bacteria may compete with the bacteria that is susceptible to the viral infection; thus reducing chances of being infected by the virus or indirectly by increasing IgA antibody production.[7] The following will help your gut break down food. They also may contain substances that block the ability of the virus to replicate. you can ferment any vegetable. (See RECIPES, Appendix A.)

- Beans are a great source of protein but if you have any dental decay sprout them first.
- Grains, Beans, Nuts and Seeds contain phytic acid (storage form of Phosphorus) that degrades when sprouted.
- Miso, Tempeh, Sauerkraut, Kimchi, Gorgonzola Cheese, Non-dairy or Dairy yogurt (if it's from raw milk and not pasteurized as the heat destroys good bacteria), Kefir.
- Olives, Pickles.

In cultures where people live to be centurions the major factor seems to be munching on fermented foods daily.

However live "culture" is available in capsules if you don't eat a lot of the above.

Probiotic capsules come in different strains. The most common and most popular and the most useful is *Lactobacillus acidophilus.* It is acid and bile resistant to survive the digestive tract and produces a lot of lactase, helpful for people with allergies to lactic acid in dairy. Some formulas contain two, three, up to twelve types of bacteria. There is a question that having more is not necessarily better—where have you heard that before—that in fact the different strains will fight, compete with each other but I'll let the researchers figure that one out. I think the best thing to do is start with a reputable brand and do your own testing.

DIFFERENT TYPES OF BENEFICIAL STRAINS, BESIDES L. ACIDOPHILUS INCLUDE:

- *Bifidobacterium bifidum.*
- *Lactobacillus bulgaricus.*
- Also *L. plantarum, L.casei, L.rhamnosus, B.longum* and *lactis* and *Streptococcus thermophilus* among others.
- There is one made from yeast that is a probiotic: *Saccharomyces boulardii.*

Dose: 50 billion a day if buying capsules like Lactobacillus acidophilus or Saccharomyces boulardii. However, you don't need to buy expensive probiotics that aid digestion by adding good flora to your gut if you make sure to have at least one teaspoon of fermented food daily.

Pre-biotics or FOS (fructooligosaccharide) support the viability of probiotics. They are made from indigestible carbohydrate fibers from legumes, fruit, and honey that the gut bacteria breaks down by short chain fatty acids (SCFAs) including lactic acid and butyric acid. They are found particularly in fermented foods, seaweeds, dandelion greens, and those that contain inulin (chicory root, jicama root, beets, onions, leeks, asparagus) beta glucan (oats, barley), pectin (apples) or glucomannan (konjac root).

ENZYMES

Enzymes are microscopic molecules responsible for almost all chemical reactions in your body. Some help digest food and some digest the waste that builds up in the bloodstream. If there are not enough enzymes to do either of these tasks then you can feel tired, headachy, sluggish etc. while the blood continues to amass undigested food particles and decayed cells. These then interfere with oxygen transfer and the natural detoxification process as well as other metabolic processes. This leads to dampening down the immune system, decreasing flexibility in the joints (where toxins love to gather), increasing pain or at least making you feel run down, tired. As we get older, we lose the ability to make HCl, hydrochloric acid as well as digestive enzymes.

FOODS WITH POSITIVE ELEMENTS

See "Optimal Grocery List" in Chapter 13

POLYPHENOLS AND FLAVONOIDS

Polyphenols are rich in antioxidants that decrease inflammation, lubricate mucus membranes and free up congestive airways. Flavonoids are a type of polyphenol that are richest in fruit peels. There are other sub-groups including sulforaphane, resveratrol and tannins. You must get these from the following foods, not from supplements:

- Black, Green and White Tea
- Black Elderberries, Blackcurrants, Berries (all kinds) Sweet Cherries, Plums, Pomegranate
- Flaxseed meal
- Artichokes
- Hazelnuts
- Most Herbs and Spices

CAFFEIC ACID

Caffeic acid contains a lot of polyphenols. It's not only anti-inflammatory but has been shown to inhibit the growth of influenza A virus in vitro, particularly in the early stages of infection,[8] and is implicated in inhibiting COVID-19 (as per chapter on COVID-19). It is in the following foods:

- Fruits – Apples, Pears, Strawberries
- Vegetables – Cabbage, Cauliflower, Kale, Olives, Mushrooms, Radishes
- Herbs – Basil, Thyme, Oregano, Sage, Turmeric
- Miscellaneous - Bee Propolis, Olive oil
- NRF2 (Nuclear factor erythroid 2-related factor 2)

This molecule is involved in the liver's Phase ll of detoxification. It regulates antioxidants and enzymes through flavonoids and other phenolic compounds. It is known to decrease oxidative stress by 40% in 30 days thereby increasing resistance to disease. It also supports mitochondrial function.[9] In:

- Fruits - Apples, Berries, Grapes, Citrus particularly Lemons, Grapefruit, Oranges
- Vegetables - Yellow onion, Scallions, Broccoli, Celery, Green Beans, Hot Pepper
- Legumes - Chickpeas, Mung Beans
- Herbs - Parsley, Thyme
- Misc. - Red Wine, Green, Black and White Teas and Chocolate

FOODS HIGH IN SULFORAPHANE

These foods are sulfur rich and include amino acids, methionine or cysteine[10]:

- Fruit - Peaches, Apricots
- Vegetables - Onions, Garlic, Green Leafy Vegetables especially Brassicaceae family except kale (often toxic in thallium), Asparagus
- Seafood (not recommended because of high levels of mercury, except sardines and occasionally wild salmon.)
- Meat – Turkey, Chicken, Beef (make sure to buy organic and/or grass fed), Eggs
- Legumes - Black Beans, Chickpeas, Lentils, Kidney Beans, Soybeans (fermented like tempeh only)
- Grains - Oats, Teff, Wild Rice, Quinoa
- Seeds – Pumpkin, Sesame
- Nuts – Brazil nuts, Almonds, Walnuts

NLRP3 INFLAMMASOMES INHIBITORS

To expand on what was discussed in Chapter 3 regarding inflammasomes, the NLRP3 inflammasome is a critical component of the innate immune system[11]. It enhances the proinflammatory cytokines IL-1 and IL-18 in response to a viral (or other microbial) infection and cellular damage. Also, as observed earlier, pro-cytokines are important in moderation but with our toxic environment, as mentioned, this process can wing out of control. We've spoken about Vitamin C and D being able to calm a cytokine storm. Now we add foods[11] with bona fide research that was unavailable when I started practice in 1987!

So many foods or food ingredients inhibit or regulate NLRP3 inflammasomes, including:

- Green tea
- Curcumin in both Turmeric and Ginger
- Propolis
- Quercetin
- Resveratrol (red wine and grape skins)
- Ginseng
- Mango
- Aloe Vera
- Jasmine
- Sulforaphanes

Some of these activate NFkB and nitric oxide (NO). It's no wonder eating a healthy diet is crucial to hindering a cytokine storm!

MELATONIN

You most likely know Melatonin as a sleep inducer, but it acts beyond the control of circadian rhythm. Doris Loh in her review article cited in Chapter 7: "The fact that the pro-inflammatory cytokine storm effects are induced by the activation of NLRP3 inflammasomes, the ability of melatonin to INHIBIT NLRP3 inflammasome elevates this powerful molecule to a truly unique position in the fight against COVID-19." Other studies confirm it plays an incredible role in a COVID-19 treatment plan. Thus, there is so much less chance of developing acute lung disease and a cytokine storm.

MORE GOOD FOOD COMPONENTS

TRYPTOPHAN

Through its relation with the NT (neurotransmitter), serotonin, is found in:

- Dairy products (milk, low-fat yogurt, cheese); Poultry (turkey, chicken); Seafood (shrimp, salmon, halibut, tuna, sardines, cod)
- Nuts and seeds (flax, sesame, pumpkin, sunflower, cashews, peanuts, almonds, walnuts)
- Legumes (kidney beans, lima beans, black beans split peas, chickpeas)
- Fruits (apples, bananas, peaches, avocado)
- Vegetables (spinach, broccoli, turnip greens, asparagus, onions, seaweed)
- Grains (wheat, rice, barley, corn, oats)

B6

Converts Tryptophan into Melatonin yielding:

- Bananas; Dried Prunes; Avocado; Spinach; Sunflower Seeds; Flax; Pistachio Nuts; Fish (tuna, salmon, halibut); Lean Beef; Chicken

CALCIUM

Helps our brain make Melatonin, so:

- Dark Leafy Greens; Green Snap Peas; Broccoli; Cauliflower; Brussels Sprouts; Almonds; Figs; Chia Seeds

NITRIC OXIDE (NO)

These foods are high in NO or convert to NO (see Chapter 7, COVID-19):

- Pomegranate
- Watermelon
- Beets
- Garlic
- Leafy Greens
- Meat: Beef, Poultry and Seafood
- Nuts and Seeds
- Dark Chocolate

OMEGA THREES

One of the strongest anti-inflammatories and the important fatty acid found in:

- Fish (wild salmon and halibut, sardines)
- Walnuts
- Chia seeds
- Hemp seeds

Dosage varies from 250 mg a day to over ten times that depending on needs. (Thus, the importance of working with an integrated health professional.) Recent research shows the importance of essential fatty acids as a contributor to infection resolution.[12]

VITAMINS

Vitamins and minerals are essential building blocks for healthy immune function. They help lymphocyte activation and proliferation, T-helper cell differentiation and many others to strengthen our immune processes, our resistance to disease.

Since our soil is depleted it's a great idea to check your unique micronutrient levels through a reputable lab and supplement. Or simply take a high quality multi vitamin and mineral with trace minerals daily. They are water soluble, so you can't take too much as you will pee any extra out.

At the top of the list is our revered favorite Vitamin C. All the way back to 1950s Vitamin C was shown to reduce symptoms and the length of illness as well by decimating viruses.

Any pathogenic virus increases oxidative stress in the body, *i.e.* molecules have been oxidized, their electrons taken away. Vitamin C, as an antioxidant, quenches these free radicals by donating electrons. This is the disease process and is what makes a toxin whether virus, bacteria, or heavy metal and so on toxic. It's clawing away at the body, building up oxidative products. When the body has enough antioxidants to donate electrons and stop this oxidation process, healing occurs. There are lots of good antioxidants, but Vitamin C is small and is able to get into all tissues especially if it is liposomal, meaning it's made to be fat soluble.

Vitamin C is known to eradicate all viruses. As seen, it reduces oxidative stress; regulates hypoxia signaling, supports mitochondrial and modulates immune defenses to stem the progression of cytokine storms. It enhances nitric oxide (NO), increases bioavailability, synthase, and production… It can inhibit NLRP3 inflammasomes, decreasing IL-1□ secretion without inducing cytotoxic effects or cell death. Loh believes, (see Chapter 7) "Thus, the combined use of melatonin and ascorbic acid may prove to be most effective in the treatment for COVID-19 patients, especially those with cardiovascular and hypertension comorbidities."

You can get it in the following fruit and vegetables,

intravenously (see Appendix D) or in various pill forms:

- Oranges, Lemons, Guava, Grapefruit, Papaya, Cantaloupe, Kiwi, Strawberries
- Broccoli, Cauliflower, Brussels Sprouts and Peppers
- IV (intravenous) Vitamin C if needed.
- Sustained release.
- or liposomal 250 – 500 mg three times a day or more added to good multi (see Resources)

VITAMIN A

Remember the measles: severe cases have a Vitamin A deficiency; it helps the body to produce immunoglobulins (IgA), essential in healing; keeps mucus membranes moist. Unlike Vitamin C, it is fat soluble and high in:

- Sweet potatoes, carrots, apricots, cantaloupe, spinach, collards.
  You should also know:
- It can be toxic in supplements, so stay low - 25,000 IU is very safe, even for people with liver disease.
- Can be combined with beta-carotene, a precursor to Vitamin A. To avoid any threat to toxicity, especially to oncology (cancer) patients, talk to your oncologist.

VITAMIN B COMPLEX INCLUDING B12

They all do so much, including playing a crucial role in production of antibodies.

VITAMIN D

A first defense in the function of the immune system.

- Better than a flu shot and far safer!
- Can decrease a cytokine storm!
- Impacts both the innate and the adaptive immune response.
- Transforms from the inactive metabolite 25 (OH) D into active form in T and B cells, also in endothelial cells lining the upper

and lower respiratory tract.

Also be aware:

- Elimination pathway can be suppressed when medicines are taken like ibuprofen (Motrin and others), aspirin, acetaminophen (Tylenol) to stop the fever; however, Vitamin D is completely the opposite![13]
- Make sure to know your Vitamin D levels…they should be between 50 and 80. Best to get it from the sun but Vitamin D3 in caps if in a sunless northern climate.
- CAUTION: Vitamin A and D are codependent on each other to help the immune system to work properly.[14] However, do not take them together as they compete for absorption in the gastro-intestinal tract.
- There is a reverse relationship between Vitamin D concentrations and IBD, Type 1 Diabetes, MS, RA, autoimmune thyroiditis.[13] Th1 is central to many bacteria and viral infections, but if uncontrolled, can lead to autoimmune.

VITAMIN E

A potent antioxidant that neutralizes tissue and cell damage, found in:

- Vegetable Oils, Green Leafy Vegetables, Wheat Germ, Broccoli, Nuts.

VITAMIN K

Helps in clotting blood, preventing excess loss of blood. It is also helpful in blood sugar regulation, found in:

- Dark Green Leafy Vegetables, Raw Spinach and Lettuce, Cauliflower, Broccoli, Olive Oil.

ADDITIONAL FOODS AS IMMUNE ENHANCERS

BETA GLUCANS

One of the big names in immunity these days are beta glucans. These are sugars (polysaccharides) in the cell walls of bacteria, fungi, yeasts, algae (seaweed), lichens and plants like brewer's yeast, oats, barley and mushrooms. Strings of glucose molecules are absorbed through the intestines, and also benefit the good bacteria.

Beta glucans are said to be the most studied as well as the most effective of all natural compounds to enhance immune function in humans.[15,16] They work through macrophages, the white blood cells (produced by the bone marrow) that patrol the body like PacMan™ men looking for foreign invaders to engulf and destroy. Macrophages have receptors that recognize beta glucans and so stimulate the immune system against viral antigens.

Bottom line is that if you ingest beta glucans your resistance to infection is amplified.

Beta glucans have been shown to be active in swine flu (H1N1)![15] and avian flu (H5N1)![15] They reduce damage to lung tissue through increasing production of interferon as well as reducing viral replication.

What is shocking and deplorable is that this has been known since the 1990s! Of course, Big Pharma doesn't make a lot of money from the inexpensive foods beta glucans are derived from. No potential profits, no investment into this possible life saving solution.

Thankfully, the U.S. Army was paying attention and in 2004 shared their research that beta glucans were the most effective immune booster of over 100 other substances they studied. Protecting humans against infection from bacteria, viruses, and fungi they also conferred protection against radiation injury![13]

The richest sources of beta glucans are baker's and brewer's yeast (*Saccharomyces cerevisiae*), oats and mushrooms.

COLOSTRUM (FERMENTED BEST)

As the first substance to be produced by the mammary gland within 72 hours of a female giving birth, colostrum is an excellent antiviral prophylactic. Prevention of Influenza Episodes with Colostrum, a study by medical doctors in Italy showed that colostrum had a significantly higher rate of decreasing numbers of flu episodes than vaccines especially in elderly patients with cardiovascular disease.[17]

Human colostrum has the main immunoglobulin as IgA whereas bovine is IgG. IgA is perfect for human babies but as we grow older our immune systems respond better to IgG, hence the use of colostrum from cows.[18]

Besides an essential source of proteins, fats, carbohydrates, minerals and vitamins, colostrum as well as contains several biologically active molecules needed for immunity; bovine colostrum contains antibodies for *E. coli, Salmonella, Streptococcus, Heliopactor pylori,* Candida and other common pathogens; also insulin growth factor I, lactoferrin and lactoperoxidase, complement factors and oligosaccharides, all components that increase the capability of our immune system by increasing passive immunity. It also contains cytokines, interferon-y, interleukin1B, Il-6 and tumor necrosis factor that can stimulate production of antibodies that neutralize hemagglutinin and neuraminidase on the virus surface!

Colostrum is virtually free of side effects. It has been shown to successfully treat acute and chronic diarrhea, and upper respiratory infections with a high dose of colostrum due to these immunoglobulins. For prevention, the dose can be much lower.

PHYTOPLANKTON: OCEAN VEGETABLE

Phytoplankton is an ocean vegetable similar to land plants. Requiring sunlight to grow and containing chlorophyll this microscopic marine plant, a microalgae, is the foundation of aquatic food webs. In a stable ecosystem jellyfish, shrimp, snails and whales are just a few ocean creatures that depend on phytoplankton for food.

There is no research to suggest phytoplankton kills the influenza virus. What it does do is kick-start your immune system. High in SOD (superoxide dismutase) considered the Queen of antioxidants, phytoplankton is able to absorb and then expel damaging free radicals, and having every mineral and amino acid needed for optimal health, as well as omega threes, phytoplankton is able to oxygenate your blood, boost your immune system through its complete nutritional profile.[19] This means an increased resistance to infection.

One of the properties of phytoplankton is to help break down foodstuffs, thereby adding to a positive gut milieu. Smaller than a red blood cell hence it is easily absorbed, making it a non-issue in one of the major problems in taking any substance: its absorption capability.

Created on land in a controlled facility there is no worry of environmental toxins that can stem from ocean garbage or from increased nutrients from pollution that can force phytoplankton to form algae blooms that can produce extremely toxic substances. Filtered ocean water runs through tubes where it reproduces continuously. By three months it becomes dark with a consistency of ketchup. Only moisture is removed (to 3 to 4%, nothing else is added) by freeze-drying and then it is ground into powder.

Dosage is a dime-sized amount of the powder mixed in water once a day, either in the morning or early afternoon. Caution: Contains Vitamin K so it is not recommended for those taking blood thinners.

MUSHROOMS

Mushrooms are not created equally, but, poisonous ones aside, they all offer something in various amounts to benefit the immune response – fiber, B vitamins, Vitamin D, minerals, amino acids, anti-inflammatory and anti-microbial and more.[20] Even the common ones, referred to as White Button that comprise ninety percent of those consumed, contain huge benefits - potassium, selenium, B vitamins and increase production of T cells that recognize and destroy toxic substances. The shiitake, maitake, reishi, cordyceps, oyster, and crimini varieties are of beta glucans. In addition, a list of beneficial ingredients in the edibles include:

- Shiitake – Vitamin D 2, 3 and 4
- Lentinen – antiviral
- Porcini - high in glutathione
- Portobello – high in riboflavin and L-ergothioneine that reduces chronic inflammatory disease
- Chanterelle – high in B vitamins, antimicrobial
- Oyster – benzaldehyde – antibacterial, anti-inflammatory
- Morels – potent anti-inflammatory
- Crimini – These help white blood cells be more active through polysaccharides; helps counter fatigue
- Enoki – Japanese – contain RIP (ribosome inactivation protein); one activity of RIP is antiviral.
- Add to broths and soups

MINERALS

Trace minerals include:

- boron, copper, iodine, iron, manganese, molybdenum, selenium and zinc
- Make sure your multi includes trace minerals or take phytoplankton.

Iodine:

- Know your level, especially if you have hypothyroidism, or Hashimotos.
- Thyroid conditions and disease are poorly treated - taking Iodoral® that has both iodine and iodide boosts the immune system and counters radiation coming from Japan. Iodide alone is said to convert as needed to iodine.

Magnesium: the most abundant mineral in the body:

- A cofactor in immunoglobulin synthesis, immune cell adherence, and so on.
- IV magnesium is used to improve lung function with people with asthma.
- Magnesium has a calming effect.
- The powder in water can be sipped on when sick.

Selenium: powerful mineral for the immune system:

- Essential for conversion of T4 to T3 in thyroid conditions, both hypo and hyper.
- Often an overlooked mineral in defense and treatment of infections.
- An absolute must-have supplement for immunological health and disease prevention and to ensure the virus does not mutate during the infection.[21]
- Take 200 IUs or 2 Brazil nuts/day.

Silver: this valuable mineral has extraordinary anti-microbial properties:[22-23]
- *The Drinkable Book* is brilliant - its pages contain nanoparticles of silver or copper to be used by countries that have bad water.
- It can be used in the case of influenza, according to some people, exclusively because of its anti-viral properties.[19,20]
- Colloidal silver is not as effective as straight silver.

Zinc: an essential mineral in any viral infection:
- Zinc has T-and B-lymphocyte activity as well as other essential activities to have a functioning immune system.
- It is also important for the thyroid.
- For prevention - 25 mg/ a day.
- Lozenges: some say they must be sucked and take no longer than a week. I've ignored that for years.
- You might need to go up to 100 mg for a week. Definitely not longer than two weeks.

KNOW YOUR FOOD ALLERGIES

Your immunity can be lowered by reactions to common allergens like peanuts, citrus, eggs, chocolate or ones unique to you like garlic or pineapple. It is important to understand that allergic foods are particular to each of us. For example, you may not have celiac disease per se, but you may have non-celiac gluten sensitivity. This means that simply by the sheer size of the gluten molecule (large) the gut rebels. This can lead to headaches, nausea, fatigue, acid reflux, itchy skin; an inflammatory reaction.

Foods that stimulate an immediate response are called IgE (Immunoglobulin E) reactions. Reactions that can take up to 72 hours to occur—Ig G or Delayed Hypersensitivity—are more confusing because you can't know what food over three days has caused this. This is why it is so important to have these food allergy tests done before you become ill if you have symptoms of almost any sort to measure your immune response to specific foods.

FOODS TO AVOID

1. Allergies: any foods showing up in IgE or IgG testing or other testing done through a reputable lab. See your integrated primary care physician (iPCP) *i.e.* naturopathic or integrated medical doctor, chiropractor, osteopath, acupuncturist or holistic nutritionist.
2. Refined sugars: be cautious of any sweetener including agave syrup. Maple syrup and rice bran syrups are okay but only on occasion. Stevia and monk fruit are best.
3. Dairy: acidic and phlegmy…not something you want when you may be about to fight a respiratory infection. Many humans are lactose intolerant; we don't make the enzyme needed to break down lactose. Dairy also contains casein, a protein that can be allergic and inflammatory. Fermented dairy products may be fine for you.
4. Non-fermented soy products: these contain protease inhibitors that turn off protein digestion. This can cause gastric upset of bloating, gas and can affect the optimization of the immune system, especially the thyroid gland.
5. Limit the nightshade family. Tomatoes, white potatoes, peppers, and eggplant; these contain solanine which is inflammatory.

LEAKY GUT SYNDROME

Be aware of leaky gut syndrome. Allergic or inflammatory foods and conditions, antibiotics, environmental toxins cause the microvilli in the gut to become inflamed, damaged. This causes undigested food to cross over into the bloodstream creating havoc.

ALKALIZE

Most vegetables and fruits are alkaline. Try alkaline water to balance out the acidity that comes with being ill.[1] Foods that are inherently acidic like dairy and wheat and other grains or anything with simple sugars should be avoided.

EXERCISE

Exercise will help keep the digestive tract and immune system strong by moving lymph and helping absorption.

ASSIGNMENT #11

1. Why is a healthy lymphatic system and gut important in healing?
2. Why is eating fermented food important? What does it supply the gut?
3. Name five foods that boost the immune system, name why.
4. How does melatonin help?

CHAPTER 12: PSYCHOLOGICAL CONSIDERATIONS

Anxiety and depression have increased significantly in the last few decades in the general population, more so since 9/11 but now in the summer of 2020 the whole country, dealing with both COVID-19 and the protests against police killings of black men, while the economy tanks, has left very few without trauma.

To learn breath work, yoga, meditation, visualization, martial arts, and have creative pursuits such as writing, dancing and singing can really help an agitated brain. Some people dispel unwanted energy by going for a bike ride or horseback riding. When you are sick in bed you are left only with your own monkey mind and that is what this brief chapter is about.

ATTITUDE

Attitude is simply re-framing a bad situation. Prayer or meditative thought is a good place to start. If you are squeamish about prayer think about it more as focusing your attention on the same consciousness that allows you to sleep, to dream, to heal cuts and wounds, that grows your hair, that deeper constant that keeps you breathing…the homeostasis of your body that is always moving forward, always trying the best it can, until your last breath.

The easiest is faking a smile and thinking of all the good things in your life. Gratitude is a great attitude changer. But this is not meant as a way to suppress any ideas or action to help heal the world. This book is about healing you and your loved ones in an acute viral infection.

BREATH WORK

Learning to control anxiety, a rapid heart rate, and any fear starts with engaging the breath rhythmically. Four breaths in, hold for four, out for four, hold for four OR four inhales and eight inhales…keep doing it for a couple minutes. This alone creates a deep positive effect on every circuit in the body. It engages the parasympathetic nervous system allowing us to feel relaxed, peaceful, letting any healing that is needed to have a chance.

VISUALIZATION

So there you are, lying in bed feeling like complete crap…you have tried to change your attitude and you have engaged your breath, now you need a deeper connection to your imagination.

Picture yourself in a beautiful environment—a mountaintop, a lake, the seashore. Allow the sound of a gentle warm breeze blowing, feel it on your skin...add gorgeous scents, perhaps lavender, sage, add the sound of water falling, perhaps some birds singing in a treetop overhead…breathe deeply in and out...let tension dissolve into the sound and images.

ADAPTED FROM MY BOOK TRANSFORMING TRAUMA[1]

The fear surrounding the time of COVID-19, and I imagine any epidemic or pandemic, is very real but usually not helpful in recovery. What it does do is focus us on feelings both that were there before an event where we felt a lack of control and were simply uncomfortable or all the way to terrified AND the fact we may not be implementing all the steps we need to in the present time. It's probably a bit of both. Whatever is going on our amygdala - fear center of the brain has been activated - and we need to pay attention, kindly to ourselves...so as not to make matters worse.

Meditation, breath work, yoga or gentle exercise can help tremendously but if you have monkey mind which is totally normal if you are sick or someone you love is sick you may want to go deeper using your five senses - imagery/sight, sound/hearing, smell, taste, touch, and your intuition and imagination. These become gateways that connect us to our brain, to memories that can be instrumental to getting to our past truth that is infringing on the present.

We use the five senses to go back in time or alternatively to describe the present in order to relax and feel calm in this time of illness. We consciously "change the channel."

Delving into our inner realm means we are immersed in authenticity with these very trusted advisors whether our five senses and simply seeing or hearing waves gently rolling into a shore or seeing a pristine wilderness view that generates peace and safety. We also create characters including their voices, we can imagine they are there with us...like a comforting grandmother even if she has long passed or never existed. They can tell a truth, they can confirm an experience or create one, bringing it to the now to soothe. And normally, in my experience, we don't need to worry; using the senses to visualize our inner world will give us only what we can bear, or process.

This approach begins with simple visualization, engaging what the mind's eye sees and layer it with the other four senses to get an even more 3D experience. And, to repeat, we can keep it very simple by creating a place of peace for you or a loved one.

Children are really good at this. You can add a softly sung song for further distraction from the discomfort of the infection or generate tranquility. This is a good time to use an essential oil in the room like lavender or ylang ylang.

Visualization, repeated and focused, is a very direct way of using thought to stimulate neurons aka neurostimulation. Brain scans show blood rushing to visual neurons that are being activated. This area of the brain is the posterior lobe; it normally processes both pain and visual perception. Constantly doing it prevents the lobe from processing pain.

TRACKING

Tracking in most acute illness like an epidemic or pandemic, in my opinion, needs to be gentle and not as a way to dig into deeper past pain. We are dealing with an acute condition and must focus on the physical. Once a person is well, then you can probe the mind-body connection and deeper truths. Right now, you want to soothe anxiety and/or fear.

The first thing to do is acknowledge the anxiety, thank it for helping to protect, to help you see the situation more closely. You can imagine bringing flowers or other beautiful meaningful objects to it. You are understanding its presence...

The left brain is great at organizing but you can't just think away psychological trauma, you have to feel it if only to see and feel or taste it at a distance and bring it flowers. This is your way to transform difficult emotions.

- **Tracking Steps:**
  1. Begin by having you or the person you're treating visualize the five senses—smell, taste, texture, sight and hearing. For instance:
     a. Sight - seeing a place, as on a mountaintop or in a meadow.
     b. Sound - add the sound of branches in a breeze.
     c. Touch - feel the soft earth or a flower.
     d. Smell - smell the forest.
     e. Taste - this is often a taste from an enjoyable memory.
  2. Taking all five senses we create a place of peace where we can begin to discover what else is there. Create a safe space in the mind's eye - beach, mountain top...if the person can't see it tell them to pretend... (works every time).
  3. Call forward the full potential self - have the person see or feel that part of themselves that is behind the conscious mind, the healer or wise person within. Some religious people will use their symbolism or people.
  4. Make sure they are committed to the process. Have them say: "I am committed to this process of healing."
  5. Now it's time to probe fear's positive intent. Acknowledge that fear is a layer of protection.
  6. Create a place of peace. Feel calm like a wave rolling into the shore.

ASSIGNMENT #12

1. What techniques can you use to help someone feel calmer?
2. Choose one and discuss in depth.
3. Do you have a favorite and why?

PART FOUR: PRACTICAL APPLICATION WITH PROTOCOLS

This final part focuses on practical procedures in order to optimize you and your family, or your patients' health through prevention as well as treatment under normal conditions. We start with prevention, with no pathogenic virus on the horizon, move to a place where and when conditions become more stressed and deeper prevention is needed, *i.e.* when a viral infection is beginning to cause harm in the community, and then focus on the sick room should you or a loved one experience an active outbreak. The last chapter will offer advice on the aftermath, what to do after the illness has taken its toll, as many people say they have never been well since experiencing an infectious disease. Or it took a long time to recover which will especially be true for anyone who experienced a ventilator while ill.

Many of the listed applications can be implemented any time, of course, as the goal is to boost the immune system. What has come before, the last three parts in this book, will give you a firm foundation, an understanding of the rationality of the ensuing recommendations and protocols. But if that's not your thing you can take my word for it and simply follow the protocols.

CHAPTER 13: PREVENTION

The basis of true prevention is good nutrition[1]—nutrient dense and anti-inflammatory with added supplements, herbs, lifestyle modifications such as exercise and a daily detox, along with still point therapy such as meditation, yoga, exercise and a creative outlet to engage the five senses as discussed in chapter 12. All aspects of being human must be considered: the physical, the psychological, the connection to each other and the earth. (Loneliness is a huge factor especially now in COVID-19, and especially with the elderly. Consider reaching out, ask them if you can get them something at the store, take out their garbage. Connection can dispel the feeling of helplessness that then depresses the immune system.)

Take the time to get all your ducks in order. Feel what's appropriate for you and/or your family. It's best to find a naturopathic physician (ND or NMD) or other integrated or functional health professional (MD, DC, DO), all referred here on in as iPCP (Integrated Primary Care Physician/Provider) that you feel comfortable with and who can get to know you and your family ideally before any sickness emerges. Alternatively, find a health care provider who is holistic or integrated, a well-trained homeopath, herbalist, traditional naturopath, nurse practitioner or physician's assistant who practices in acute situations. You may also need a holistic psychologist or psychotherapist if you have had any kind of trauma. It depends. (I practice naturopathic medicine, am board certified in homeopathy and practice creative psychotherapy.) Hopefully you have a good sense of what an appropriate health care provider brings to the table.

Ask your health professional if they make house calls.

This is the time to order your supplies:

1. Homeopathic kit (see Resources. Add the COVID-19 nosode to this.) This needs to be available whether you are self-treating (make sure you've gained knowledge) or waiting for your homeopath whether ND, MD or other to prescribe. You don't want to have to wait for it to come in the mail or even go out to a nearby store.
2. Botanical medicine as discussed.
   - *Lomatium*, licorice or elderberry are best for flu and licorice for COVID-19 unless the person has high blood pressure, then you will want Ashwagandha or possibly *Scutellaria*.
   - Explore herbal adaptogens (See Botanical chapter) to add a nonspecific response to your immune system.
   - Add detoxifying herbs by having teas such as Nettles, Dandelion root, Burdock, Cinnamon available.
3. Basic Supplements: (dosage to be determined by body weight and lab work)
   - Melatonin, Vitamin C (preferably liposomal), glutathione[2] are essential.
   - Daily sun or if this is not possible, Vitamin D.
   - Phytoplankton is another must to start taking daily. Also, Zinc.
4. Labs. This is best addressed with your iPCP. Definitely Vitamin D, Iron (Fe), Hemoglobin (Hb), and possibly C-reactive protein (CRP) for general inflammation. This is the time to check your food allergies - IgE and IgG; mineral levels and ratios and heavy metals through a hair analysis company (see Resources) and if you can, check your toxins further through GPL or Doctors Detox. There are so many tests that may be warranted, *i.e.* hormones or genetics. Ask your iPCP.

A WORD ON UNDERLYING CONDITIONS

An underlying condition and therefore a weakened immune system can generate especially severe symptoms with a pathogenic virus.

Most at risk, whether child or adult, are:

- the elderly.
- those with asthma, chronic lung, heart, kidney disease, obesity or diabetes.

- drug addicts.
- the homeless.
- the emotionally fragile.
- someone immunocompromised from chemotherapy or steroid treatment.

Get to work to heal these as best as you are able. Don't do it alone. Find the right professional(s) to work with depending what's going on. Here is an example of how to address asthma:

- Test delayed-sensitivity food allergies.
- Determine vitamin and mineral status.
- Keep the home free of dust and mold.
- Add colostrum or aloe or phytoplankton daily to boost the gut (where the immune system is most active).
- Take a good probiotic and a good multivitamin or phytoplankton.
- Hydrate.
- Address the emotional basis, the body-mind connection (often fear in asthma) to get to the root of the condition.

Now let's start with what you can do at home to get your immune system in the best possible shape.

NUTRITION

This optimal grocery list is everything discussed in the book. All food must be organic or at least pesticide free from a farmer's market. Present environmental conditions affect the quality of our soil and make organic vegetables and fruits essential. (If you are unconvinced, see Chapter 5, The Burden of Toxins, specifically glyphosate, pesticides, and heavy metals.) Even as a single mother with extremely little money I found a way to buy organic. I know I am a health nerd, and my daughter has many funny stories about her experience, but this is one aspect of motherhood in which I have no regrets.

OPTIMAL GROCERY LIST

- Fruits – Apples, Apricots, Bananas, Berries of all kinds, Cantaloupe, Citrus - Lemons, Grapefruit and Oranges, Coconut,

Figs, Grapes, Peaches, Pears, Pomegranate, Prunes, Strawberries, Tart Cherries, Watermelon.

- Vegetables – Asparagus, Avocado, Beets, Broccoli Sprouts, Brussels Sprouts, Broccoli, Cabbage, Cauliflower, Celery, Cucumber, Dark leafy greens (Arugula, Burdock, Dandelion), Garlic, Green Beans, Green Snap Peas, Hot Peppers, and Leeks, Medicinal Mushrooms (Cordyceps, Reishi, Shitake), Olives, Onion, Peas, Radishes, Parsley, Olives, Seaweed, Spinach, Scallions.
- Legumes - Black Beans, Chickpeas, Lentils, Lima Beans, Mung Bean Sprouts, Split Peas, Soybeans (fermented like Tempeh only).
- Fermented Foods - Kefir, Kimchi, Miso, Olives, Pickles Sauerkraut, Tempeh, Yogurt (non-dairy).
- Grains – Almost anything sprouted; Oats, Wild Rice, Quinoa, Rice, Barley, Teff.
- Nuts and Seeds - Brazil Nuts, Chia Seeds, Flax Seeds, Hemp Seeds, Pistachios, Pumpkin Seeds*, Sesame Seeds, Sunflower Seeds*, Walnuts. (*sprouted is best)
- Fish (if desired) - Seafood has high levels of mercury. Sardines, Wild Salmon (occasionally), Halibut, and Mackerel.
- Meats – Beef, Turkey, Chicken (organic/grass fed only).
- Eggs – organic only.
- Herbs – (Almost all will be high in antioxidants.) Turmeric, Basil, Bay Leaf, Cardamom, Chili Seeds, Cinnamon, Cumin, Fennel, Ginger, Marjoram, Mustard Seeds, Oregano, Rosemary, Sage, Thyme.
- Oils – Coconut, Olive.
- Miscellaneous – Phytoplankton, Bee Pollen and Propolis (from your area and guaranteed pesticide free), Coconut butter (for MCTs, good for brain).
- Teas – *Cistus incanus*, Black, Green and White, Dandelion, Ginger, Mint, Nettle, *Tulsi* (Holy Basil), Rhodiola, Chicory, and many more.
- Sweetener – Monk Fruit, Stevia, Coconut Sugar, Medicinal Raw Honey (from an unpolluted source).
- Add herbs and spices to your cooking on a daily basis and drink 2-3 cups of tea a day (see above and change them up) to keep the immune system ready for any bug that comes along.
- Stock up on clean, preferably alkaline, water.

- See RECIPES, Appendix A.

FAMILY PREVENTION TIME

The flu season (with or without COVID-19) usually starts in the fall often around the time children are going back to school. For families, while this may not be the best time to start the described preventive protocols that follow as life can become extremely busy with schoolwork and after school activities after a leisurely summer, just do your best, don't beat yourself up. Slowly introduce better nutritional practices and health habits and you may be surprised to discover that you may well be able to prevent or decrease the onset of influenza or another viral infection like COVID-19 and its possible complications. If you have a family, you might want to teach them what to do just as you would teach them earthquake prevention and first aid. After school is out in late spring may be a perfect time to take the time as a family to implement what has been discussed in this book.

DECREASE YOUR TOXIC LOAD

Everyday pollutants in the air, water and food contribute further to an already dysregulated (*i.e.* dysfunctional) immune system. Although best addressed under the care of a health professional, you can begin by switching to an organic diet, reducing any synthetic drugs, chemicals in cosmetics, cleaning products and bed linens and incorporating an overall healthy toxin free lifestyle that will protect brain and body from environmental exposures.

Make sure your home and bedroom particularly are free of environmental toxins lest they augment the full-blown toxic situation albeit generated from a virus. Purchase a HEPA filter if you live in a city or town with poor air quality.

One of the biggest toxins in your bedroom is your mattress.[3] Mattresses are made with toxic foams that can release volatile compounds that wreak havoc with our endocrine and immune systems. If you can't change it, then buy a good HEPA filter; these filters also trap dust containing airborne bacteria and viruses that contribute to the possibility of becoming sick with a severe co-infection. Alternatively, open the window to increase the flow of fresh air and sunlight, both antimicrobial. Children especially are vulnerable to toxic chemicals.[4]

Again, as added protection, seek guidance from a naturopathic doctor or an expert in detoxification about your possible toxic load that can lead to a deeper dive, determining intermediary biomarkers that expose individual toxicity.

It is especially important for women to detox before they become pregnant. Toxins have the ability to cause over reactivity in children to common things such as food and pollen and are under-reactive to common pathogens such as viruses and bacteria.[5]

In the meantime, understand that the main organ of detoxification is the liver, and is amplified by dandelion (*Taraxacum officinalis*) and milk thistle (*Silybum marianum*), to name two safe botanicals. You can start these without worry as you make sure your lymph and glymph (brain lymph) system is getting a workout through a diet primarily of organic fruits and vegetables, good sleep, exercise, sunshine, adding antioxidants such as glutathione and Vitamin C, soluble fiber and binders such as activated charcoal, zeolite, modified citrus pectin, chlorella, or cilantro.

Detoxification can be simple with the use of saunas (preferably infrared) daily, fasting once a week with organic juices or it can be more complicated adding colonics, fasting, and particular nutraceuticals.

Detoxing your body of stored up toxins can comprise a normal part of your lifestyle though it requires focus. Given your living circumstances, the following protocols are a quick way to detox your body from toxins periodically without breaking your budget and compromising your time. You can undertake this as part of a daily or weekly schedule.

GENERAL DAILY DETOX PLAN

VERSION A

1. Buy organic produce as much as you can find and afford, as well as organic or non-toxic cosmetics, household cleaners, laundry detergent, dryer sheets and so on.
2. Drink filtered, not-bottled water (plasticizers disrupt the immune system).
3. Fasting: intermittent or periodic. Do a 24-hour juice fast on Saturday. Generally, celery, cucumbers, carrots, beets, apples, adding juice of lemons and ginger, will work well. You can add medium chain fatty acids in the form of coconut butter or oil or MCT oil and other supplements as discussed.
4. Sauna: preferably infrared, at least once a week, or daily if you live in an urban area or in a rural area if highly concentrated with agricultural chemicals. Not only does a sauna detoxify the body from toxins, it also boosts the immune system.
5. Consume at least 40 grams of fiber daily through fruit and vegetable intake: contain antioxidants for the immune system to function properly. Make sure you use the whole organic vegetable or fruit (other than apple seeds and pits of peaches and plums) with a Nutribullet® or Vitamix® or similar machine. Increase your intake of fermented food or take a probiotic.[6]
6. If you are anticipating a busy day you can eat a light breakfast consisting of healthy fats and protein in the morning. Then drink the juice until the next morning alternating with plenty of water to keep you hydrated and for the fiber to move through the intestines. Go to sleep early, wake up early: remember the brain detoxifies and repairs at night when we sleep.
7. Exercise: Exercising promotes up-regulation of enzymes needed for detoxification and moves the lymph. Three to five minutes on a mini trampoline is a great way to get going in the morning after drinking a glass or two of filtered, alkaline water, 12 to 16 hours after your last meal.
8. Our soil is depleted thus consume dense nutrients through food

and add supplementation (see #11) as needed for detoxification.

9. Spend as much time outdoors in green spaces as indoor air is considerably more polluted than the outdoors.
10. Learn breathing and stress reducing techniques to reduce oxidative stress.
11. A great way to start the day: Drink a big glass of alkaline water on rising, jump on a trampoline, do yoga, and then meditate.
12. Specific nutrients that protect from environmental pollution include:
    a. Vitamin C – liposomal best.
    b. Vitamin E - alpha-tocopherol.
    c. Beta-Carotene.
    d. Omega-3 fatty acids.
    e. Sulforaphanes (remember the importance of Sulfur in detoxing - foods: Broccoli and family of Crucifers).
    f. B Vitamin Complex.
    g. Iodoral® - a combination of Iodine and Iodide; if Iodine is low it will be crowded out by the Halogen family pollutants, Chlorine, Bromine and Fluoride.
    h. Zinc – needs to be balanced with copper.
    i. Glutathione.
13. Another factor to be aware of is to turn off EMFs, electromagnetic fields especially 5G. WIFI, computers, cell phones and the like affect our immune system.

VERSION B (More Specific)

1. Eat a healthy breakfast in the morning and go for an easy walk.
2. From 30 - 60 min after eating breakfast, take 20-60 minutes for a regular sauna or steam.
3. Cool off every 10-15 minutes in a cool shower to prevent overheating and to remove the toxins that have sweated out through the skin.
4. For an infrared sauna, try 15- 20 minutes, cool shower immediately after.
5. It is essential to hydrate with electrolytes before, during, and after the sauna. Drinking the juice or detox smoothie described in Version A throughout the day will aid in the detoxification process.

6. Do the same protocol for two more days. You should feel great, and sleep should come easily that night and energy the next day.
7. Optional: A colonic 12 to 24 hours later.

VERSION C (Water Fast)

1. If you do not have a busy schedule, just hang out around home and read, meditate, do yoga or gentle exercise, walk in fresh air.
2. This is a great way to remove toxins and decrease inflammation.
3. Do not combine this with a sauna as it may substantially reduce blood sugar levels causing severe hypoglycemia.
4. This kind of fast must be done under the supervision of a knowledgeable health practitioner.
5. Turn off all electronics in order to reduce distractions and the toxic effects of electromagnetic radiation.
    - Sip the following mixture every 15 minutes throughout the day for energy and detox support: Boil 1 cup of filtered water and let it cool off. Mix in up to 1 teaspoon of raw honey (from safe hives) and 1/2 of squeezed lemon to taste. Make a big jug as you will drink up to 6-8 cups per day.
    - About Colonics: Weekly colonics (colon cleansing) is one of the best ways to get rid of toxins when combined with nutrition and a sauna. Check out the late Dr. Walter Crinnion, N.D. in his book, *Clean Green and Lean*. I interned with him and formulated my own *The 35 Day Detoxification and Rejuvenation Programme*. Designed in 1988 for my Kitsilano clinic it included many colonics. Patients would come in yearly or seasonally. If you have never had one, try them. They can make a huge difference, start with a minimum of three.

A SIMPLE WEEKLY HEALTH PREVENTION PLAN

Here is a weekly prevention plan for those who are new at getting healthy and/or very busy during the week from Dr. Alec.

DAILY CALENDAR

MONDAY
(can be the most stressful day of the week) • Meditation is always helpful. • On waking, drink a cup of warm water with a fully squeezed lemon. This helps with waste elimination, blood alkalizing and immune stimulation/modulation as lemons are high in citric acid, vitamin C and copper. • If you take showers in the morning use this time for a quick boost of energy and improving immune functioning: shower 3 minutes of warm water then switch to 30 seconds of cooler, even cold, water. Repeat 3 times for a total of a 10-minute shower. Always end on Cold. This procedure will give you extra energy and stabilize the immune system for the rest of the day. • During the day try to take 5-10-minute breaks for breathing exercises, and/or gentle walking to decrease inflammation. Take your lunch outside and eat slowly, enjoying your food. If you are feeling stressed, consider listening to music in the car or on the bike or walk to work. Stress from listening or watching the (bad) news increases inflammation. When home do some exercise—even a 15-minute walk, preferably if you have one, with family. Cook and eat dinner together, read a book or anything else that brings you together. Plopping down on the couch in front of the television set to eat dinner is apparently one of the worst things you can do for your immune system, even though we all do it. • Do not forget to take your vitamins and minerals throughout the day.

- So much accumulates stress. Be careful to remain calm returning home in traffic, picking up kids who might be agitated, shopping while talking on the phone, driving to pick up your significant others etc. etc. all increases inflammation. Find time for yourself and go to sleep as early as possible (ideally by 9:00 PM) in order for your body to recover from the stressful day. The least agitated you are before sleep the deeper and more restful sleep will be.
- Take a warm shower or a bath with Epsom salts and relaxing herbs such as chamomile or lavender herbs will help.
- Reading a book or listening to music are other ways to put your body into a parasympathetic state, which will increase your recovery from the stressful Monday.
    - Ideally 6:00 PM - 7:00 PM is the best time to finish eating, and then nothing until about 7:00 AM the next day. This puts the body into the 12-hour intermittent fasting period where the body can detoxify itself from sugar and oxidative stress. Consuming high sugar foods throughout the day then not eating for 12 hours will create an early increase of cortisol at night -around 3:00 AM – 4:00 AM or earlier- causing night cravings and inability to sleep through the night. As naturopathic doctors we see an epidemic of patients waking up around 3:00 AM – 5:00 AM and not being able to go back to sleep. Cortisol and sugar are most likely to blame, both of which are implicated in sleep apnea, but that's for another book!

Look at the recipes for Monday in Appendix A to decrease inflammation and to increase calm. They can be prepped in 5 minutes and cooked in 30-60 minutes.

TUESDAY
• Depending on how much sleep you received the night before, repeat the Monday's health boosting recommendations while adding a more rigorous exercise and /or sauna therapy into your schedule. • If you can add high intensity exercise for at least 30 minutes in the morning or at night without compromising your sleep that would be ideal.

- Following exercise with water therapy and/or sauna is ideal as it decreases the inflammation created by the workout.
- If you have exercised a certain amount and the next day you are very sore or very fatigued, you have exercised too much and need to scale down to what your body can handle. Be gentle to yourself.
- Use the recipes for Tuesday in Appendix A that help with the preparation and recovery from a long day of work and exercise.

WEDNESDAY
• Check yourself in the morning: what is your energy level, how does your body and mind feel? If you are fatigued and inflamed, it might be time to slow down and recharge. • Doing gentle yoga, sauna or both is worthwhile as there are 2 and half more days before the weekend. • It might be good to increase your dose of adaptogenic herbs like Ashwagandha, Vitamin C, E, Bs, enzymatic cofactors (minerals) such as Zn, Cu, Mg, Se, Mb, Essential Fatty Acids and plant antioxidants. • This is the danger time when we reach for high fat and high sugar foods as our cortisol is spiking while our energy is decreasing and the inflammation is increasing. Eat the foods described for Wednesday to stop the cravings early in the morning and boost your energy.

THURSDAY
(Again, see how your energy, mood and inflammation are): • If your energy is up and you can handle a bit more movement, exercise in the morning or after work. • Once more, nourish your body with the foods that give energy and reduce inflammation as described.

FRIDAY
(The last day of the busy week): • You may be trying to finish things up at work and may be exhausted physically, mentally and emotionally. • This might be a great day to let it go at night and just eat healthy comfort foods and watch some TV or go out and enjoy yourself. • Try not to overindulge yourself on sweets and alcohol as it will throw off your energy for the weekend when you are actually trying to recover from the busy week. • Use the recipes for healthy desserts and choose alcohol wisely. Yes, alcohol is good for you in moderation and if combined with herbs and low glycemic juices can be a great boost to your energy and immune system. Tequila and dry red wine are good choices as well as fermented drinks (added bonus of probiotics) such as Kombucha, Ginger Beer, Sima (Finnish) and Boza (Bulgaria).

SATURDAY OR SUNDAY
• Try shopping and meal planning and do some preparation for the week on the weekend (or your days off) to save time and stress. • Consider eating raw foods that are easily prepared. A Nutribullet® or equivalent allows unique combinations of raw food with protein, providing healing and preventive benefits fast. • Incorporate steamed or baked vegetables daily, another easy step. • Spend time outdoors and in nature. Expose yourself to the sun and breathe fresh air. • If you eat poorly during the week due to lack of time at work or any other reason, try to eat super healthy during the weekend. • If you have family members you live with, involve them in meal planning, shopping and cooking. Children pick up good and bad eating habits early; show them their parents are committed to being healthy. Let the kids pitch in in the preparing and cooking process. Also saves time, once they

have the knack.

- Be consistent with supplementation.
- Exercise and use the sauna or other hydrotherapy techniques (*i.e.* cold showers) to help the immune system function optimally.
- If you do not sleep well during a busy and stressful week, sleep in as much as possible on the weekend as studies show that catch-up sleep does improve sugar regulation and decreases inflammation.

Remember recipes and tonics for building and maintaining a stellar immune system are in Appendix A.

ASSIGNMENT #13

1. Start your preparations with regard to:
   a. Food - learn to make a broth, freeze
   b. Botanicals - have them ordered
   c. Homeopathic - same
   d. Hydrotherapy - have cloths, towels, and sheets clean
2. Choose the essential oils you are drawn to and order them.
3. Choose one of the detoxes to do.
4. Become familiar with the optimal grocery list, and recipes in Appendix A.

CHAPTER 14: DEEPER PREVENTION

Once a pathogenic virus is on the move it is time to step up prevention and move into a deeper awareness of a pathogenic virus. Make sure to cover your mouth. Wash hands with warm water and soap and try to keep your hands away from your face. **DO NOT USE TOXIC PRODUCTS LIKE PUREL.** Use essential oils instead—see end of Botanicals. Remember that airborne or respiratory droplets can be directly transmitted through coughing or sneezing or from touching a surface someone infected has touched. And may also come from feces from shared plumbing.

LABS: In a viral infection, a lab can be done. A CBC (complete blood count) will show an increase or decrease in white blood cells and possibly atypical lymphs. CRP/C-reactive protein may be elevated although this marker is measuring general inflammation in the body. For the added lab for COVID-19 see chapter 7.

This is the time to make sure you are supplementing enough vitamins, minerals and other nutrients as discussed. Talk to your iPCP. All the following are needed now:

Vitamins	• Vitamin C (liposomal) • B vitamins (methyl form) • Vitamin D or sunshine
Mineral Complex	• Added Zinc - up to 90 mg (one week only then reduced to 30 mg)
Other Nutrients	• Phytoplankton • Probiotics • Mushroom powder • Glutathione (NAC)[1,2]

Food Prep	• Food (think of easy prep and keep it simple): Eat lightly. No sugar[2] or junk food. • Start making Broths whether from an Organic Meat bone or Vegan using Vegetables. (See Recipes.) • Have a fridge full of Vegetables including Mushrooms, low glycemic fruit, and healthy snacks. • Bake, roast or steam Sweet Potatoes, Carrots, Cabbage, Beets and so on.
Foods to Consume	• Garlic – decongestant, natural antibiotic, best when raw • Onions – antimicrobial • Turmeric – anti-inflammatory, antioxidants, decrease toxins
Botanicals	• *Cistus incanus* - antiviral • Elderberries for the flu – berries only. Can make syrups, teas, and tinctures • Jujubes – antimicrobial, strengthens immune system, calming • Thyme – helps cough • Marshmallow root - demulcent - sore throat
Rest and relax	• Take a bath with lavender oil and Epsom salts (can add Dead Sea Salts) and baking soda to create an alkaline environment and to kill any virus.
Exercise	• Exercise lightly – walk, yoga, don't overextend yourself…listen to your body.
Bowels	• Make sure bowels are moving …give chia or flaxseed smoothie (see Recipes).
Hydration	• Above all else hydrate!!!

In Chinese Medicine there is the concept of cooling and warming foods. I have put parentheses around those in the Optimal Grocery List (Chapter 13) that are not warming. Once the inflammasome is activated (*i.e.* sickness starts) consider the following:

- Cucumber is considered a cooling food and should not be eaten during a flu.
- Cinnamon, on the other hand, has thermal properties that are beneficial during the flu and can be consumed or bathed in.
- Ginger, garlic, honey, leeks and onions, nuts, oats, wild rice are all warming.
- Stay away from apples, asparagus, avocados, bananas, blueberries, cantaloupe, celery, citrus fruit, coconut water, zucchini. Neutral foods (and so are okay) include apricots, beets, carrots, corn, fava bean, flax seeds, green beans, lentils, peas, pineapple, raspberries, shiitake mushrooms.

DIFFERENTIATING A MORE PATHOGENIC VIRAL INFECTION FROM A SIMPLE COLD AND ALLERGIES

The flu or COVID-19 can be easily mistaken for the common cold and sometimes environmental and less often food allergies.

A cold is caused by a virus too…one of 100 different ones - usually a rhinovirus but mild and in most cases won't lead to any serious complications like pneumonia.

It's generally contagious for the first three days and usually clears up within a few more.

In contrast, allergies come from an overactive immune system. In environmental allergies, the body mistakes a usually harmless substance like dust or pollen for germs and releases histamine, causing a runny nose, swelling in your sinuses, coughing, and sneezing. The important thing to remember is that they do not cause fever.

Diagnosing food allergies is a different story entirely. They can be difficult to pinpoint without a test, and even then, it's not a hundred percent surety. There are two types: Immediate or IgE, meaning you will have a reaction very soon if not immediately on eating a certain food. If this happens often most people have a sense of what these foods are. Delayed Hypersensitivity or IgG, on the other hand, can take up to 72 hours as the immune system mounts a defense, so it's harder to figure out what it is. (This is why an elimination diet can help: you refrain from all food for a few days and then add in one food at a time every three days.)

It's important to point out that those with environmental or food allergies may be predisposed to more infections as the immune system is preoccupied with dealing with the allergy while becoming less vigilant towards infections.

PROPHYLACTICALLY WITH HOMEOPATHY

- If it may be a flu: you can take homeopathic Boiron® *Oscillococcinum* as preventive
- Or if you start feeling ill: you can take homeopathic Aconite, low dose.
- If you think it may be COVID-19: Consider the COVID-19 nosode or *Arsenicum album* / India is doing this at this time. (See Homeopathic section for more.)

A MORE STRINGENT PROTOCOL

Multi-Vitamin	• A high dose of multivitamin-mineral that contains Vitamins A, D, C, Zn, Bs, Mg, Se, Cu, N-acetyl-cysteine or continue to eat well and take Phytoplankton daily if you are otherwise feeling well.
Fish Oil	• Fish oil (high quality-be careful of rancidity) for omega threes or nightly chia seeds in water with magnesium powder.
Probiotics	• Probiotics or increase fermented foods.
Sauna	• Sauna (see Resources) 15-20 minutes daily if infrared or at least two-three times a week. • A steam bath or regular sauna as long as comfortable OR hot bath with essential oils 2-3 times per week. Make sure to hydrate before, during, and after, and cool down with a cool shower before wrapping up with blankets or clothing. • If a steam or sauna, going back and forth between hot and cool (time 3:1) can boost the immune system significantly.

Botanicals	• Immune modulating, herbal adaptogens and detoxifying teas or tinctures or in the following foods: • Reishi Mushroom and others noted • Ginger • Elderberry • Licorice • Lemon • Nettles • *Tulsi* (Basil) • Thyme • Ashwagandha root • Rhodiola rosea • Siberian ginseng root • Coriander • Cloves • Saffron - See Appendix A: Recipes

A REMINDER

As discussed in chapter 3, the first line of defense to any virus are the neutrophils that engulf and destroy pathogens. These are positively affected by glutathione[2] but negatively by acetaminophen (Tylenol). Phagocytosis decreases 2X with simple sugars like glucose, fructose, orange juice or honey. Studies have shown it can take neutrophils 5 hours to recover.

For the initial stages of the **INFLAMMASOME** being activated (starting to feel ill), make sure you are taking some form of probiotics, Vitamin A (best from food like sweet potatoes), Vitamin C (high doses like 1 gm an hour to bowel tolerance) and D (make sure to have spent time in the sun for more reasons than D like sulfur) and glutathione which can be in the form of NAC, its precursor. Minerals too but these can come from broths and smoothies.

Once you have fever means the cytokine, interferon, has recognized the virus and is coming to the rescue by enhancing T lymphocytes for the next stage of immune action. The Adaptive System which being cell-mediated will begin to eliminate the viral infected cells *i.e.* rash, cough, and will engage T lymph and T killer cells, while being positively influenced by glutathione and again negatively by acetaminophen and toxic substances like mercury.

Because of all this action with the white blood cells now generating ROS (reactive oxygen species) keep taking Vitamin C and other free radical quenchers in order to halt the virus. You will also need more than adequate Vitamin D to guard against a cytokine storm. Another positive influence is gentle exercise or a jump on a mini trampoline so your lymph system is ready to detox further. Remember—at the risk of boring you—do not take suppressive medication like acetaminophen or aspirin.

IS IT COVID-19 OR INFLUENZA?

Particulars In Influenza	• Incubation is one to two days, during which time it is infectious
	• Portals of influenza virus entry into human body:
	    • Ear
	    • Mouth
	    • Conjunctiva of eye
	    • Nose
	    • Broken skin
	    • Insect bite
	    • Organ or bone transplant
	    • Blood transfusion
	    • Placenta (pregnant females)
	    • Urethra
	    • Anus
	    • Vagina
	    • Penis

Symptoms: May Be Severe	• Stuffy or runny nose • Fever or chills • Usually Sore throat • Dry, hacking cough • Muscle aches, bone aches, headaches • Profound fatigue that can last up to three weeks • Possibly nausea and vomiting (more in children) • Sleep is often disturbed • The fever can last up to 3 days; a full recovery can take a week or longer

Particulars In Covid-19 (Sars-Co-V-2)

- Incubation is 5 - 6 days during which time it is infectious. Although unlikely there may be a pre-symptomatic period so consider it up to 14 days.
- Portals of Covid influenza virus entry into human body:
    - Nose
    - Mouth - possible
    - Conjunctiva of eye - possible
    - Symptoms (from mild to severe):
    - Fever or chills
    - Cough
    - Shortness of breath or difficulty breathing
    - Fatigue
    - Muscle or body aches
    - Headache
    - New loss of taste or smell
    - Sore throat
    - Congestion or runny nose
    - Nausea or vomiting
    - Diarrhea
- If you are worried that COVID-19 is implicated in symptoms get tested.

ALWAYS TAKE THESE BODILY PROCESSES INTO ACCOUNT

MUCUS

Yuck mucus, right? Actually no. As much as we want to get rid of excess mucus it actually is doing its best to get us well. It gets rid of the harmful wastes as noted regarding the difference between Th 1 and Th 2 immune systems. Mucus also protects us from invading pathogens and environmental irritants, coating our respiratory system to create an essential barrier.[3,4]

Mucus production increases in any respiratory condition: it

becomes thicker and more difficult to clear. The answer is not initially how do we dry this up but the questions are how can mucus move quickly through the body with its accompanying trapped particles/pathogens?

The answer is making the mucus thin and watery.

Mucus contains substances that dissolve chemical bonds thus decreasing mucus's viscosity. These agents include lysozymes (enzymes that break up bacterial cell walls), immunoglobulins (IgA) predominates (a deficiency sets up people for infections), lactoferrin (this increases ciliary action hence clearing time) and electrolytes (salts.)

There are various ways to help achieve the goal of clearing thick mucus, getting it out of the lungs and/or sinuses:

1. Drink water with lemon or herbs (see botanical section for expectorants) for electrolytes, sipping constantly. Basically, your work while sick is to remain hydrated. Dehydration results in the body shunting water from mucus production to the bloodstream making it.
2. Avoid dairy products. No studies except one showing opioid protein in milk (beta-casomorphin-7) have been shown to increase mucin, a major mucus protein.[3]
3. NAC and PI increase mucolytic activity by breaking disulfide bonds resulting in the breakdown of mucoproteins hence increasing the clearing of thick mucus: (a) N-acetylcysteine (NAC) is an amino that increases glutathione, the body's most powerful antioxidant, 500mg three times a day or 900 mg twice a day; (b) Potassium iodide (PI)[5] does this as well and also stimulates the cilia in the respiratory tract and sinuses. An added bonus is it is antimicrobial.[5]

CONSTIPATION

One needs to guard against constipation at all times, and especially during a vicious illness such as COVID-19. Constipation is most probably the body screaming to be hydrated. Constipation creates toxicity in the body by inhibiting waste from being removed, including the build-up of viral debris.

Usually the result of dehydration, constipation will decrease mucus clearing.[4]

Fiber and staying hydrated is the answer here. My favorite fiber source is soaked chia seeds although soaked flax seeds also work well.

Constipation is a byproduct of our insomniac, western diet and microbiome-disrupted environment. Constant stress alone can stop gut motility causing severe havoc on the rest of the body. Dysbiosis (gut microbiome dysregulation[5]) is one of the causes of constipation and the addition of probiotics has been shown to improve it.[6, 7]

FEVER

Once a virus is replicating in your cells, pathogenic or not, you want a high enough temperature that is beyond the bugger's ability to function. Therefore, it is essential to NOT suppress a fever. If the body temperature goes higher than 103 degrees pat down with a cool cloth or go in a cool bath or shower.

Many illness-causing pathogens prefer the body's normal temperature and a fever will mean killing the bad guys. A fever also punches up the white blood cells, our immune system fighters.

Remember, a fever is not an illness itself, it simply indicates infection. It is only one part of the picture in an illness. And for children it is an unreliable indicator of the severity of it. Many children run around with a high fever and others can be very sick with a subnormal temperature.

The benefits of fever cannot be overstated. The fever destroys the fever-causing microorganisms when exposed to higher temperatures. This is how your body, your immune system, helps you to heal.

The best is to let a fever run its course to help fight off the virus or possible secondary bacterial infection. In a viral infection the body needs to heat up to initiate a die off of the virus. Studies show that children who run a fever during their first year are less likely to develop allergies later in childhood. If the vital force or "qi" is strong then best to simply keep hydrated while resting in bed, limit food, and use cool cloths, following the basics outlined in this booklet. See below if the person's vitality or qi is low.

A fever between 99 degrees and 102 degrees is killing the bad guys. Above this the need to cool the body is usually only necessary to decrease discomfort. Good to know the brain has an internal regulatory mechanism that prevents fevers caused by infection from getting higher than 106 degrees. Only four percent of children will have fever seizures—momentary loss of consciousness, eyes rolling back, stiffening, twitching—and these cause no permanent harm. In our society, however, 103 F is the limit before seeing your doctor or going to the hospital.

The American Academy of Pediatrics does not recommend fever-reducing drugs, a huge change over the years. This is good news as studies show aspirin and ibuprofen suppress the white blood cells necessary to destroy any secondary bacterial infection in influenza. Acetaminophen (Tylenol) should never be taken for anything or by anyone due to possible liver damage.

AN ASIDE

In North America it was the indigenous people who taught the farmer turned medicine man the idea that steam heals. Samuel Thomson used the botanical *Lobelia inflata,* also known as Indian tobacco, Pokeweed and Gagroot among others, in fevers. The root is supposed to be most medicinal but leaves and stems are what Alma Hutchens states in her book *Indian Herbalogy of North America.* Otherwise is a fever a friend or foe? Same as that old joke... depends how high.

TREATMENT

First, try not to panic...It may be difficult, but it's best to do nothing or little in a minor illness. However, if you want to bring down a fever: sip cool drinks, use a fan, have a lukewarm, not cool, sponge bath. This could be the time to connect with your iPCP. Make sure they know someone in your family is getting ill.

- Homeopathic Belladonna is my favorite anti-fever... remember homeopathy does not suppress but encourages the body's innate healing.
- Diaphoretics such as Peppermint or Holy Basil (see Botanical chapter) can be given through teas to increase sweating, releasing heat through the skin, shedding toxins and waste products; use sparingly with people with low vitality.
- Another way to raise temperature in individuals who cannot mount a good temperature to fight the infection is the sauna. Saunas can safely and effectively raise the core temperature stimulating the production of white blood cells to fight the infection.[8] The biggest caution with saunas is that they can dehydrate the patient very quickly and must be done under the supervision of a knowledgeable practitioner. (See Hydrotherapy)

ASSIGNMENT #14

Instead of asking you what you'll need to get your sick room in order-dealt within the next chapter- I'll give you this heads-up:

1. Make sure the bedroom is ready in case someone becomes ill. Remember essential oils.
2. Have linens, face cloths, towels- large and small easily accessible and lots of them.
3. Organize the kitchen.
4. Make sure there is a lot of prepared broth (see Appendix A) and ingredients on hand or a smoothie.

CHAPTER 15: IN THE SICK ROOM - A VIRAL INFECTION IS ACTIVE

Once you have a diagnosis of COVID-19 or influenza proceed with caution. As a practitioner or patient, take your temperature often and put in place all that you have learned from this book. If you have been exercising all the preventive measures, taking needed nutrients, and following a daily detox with an infrared sauna, the chances are good you or your loved one will stay well. There is no guarantee. I don't know your particular genetics but from what I have experienced over the last 35 years is that natural medicine works. Beautifully.

However, given the serious nature of the present outbreak of COVID-19, proceed with caution and always stay connected to your integrated primary care provider (iPCP).

IF YOU THINK YOU HAVE PNEUMONIA

Pneumonia is what you are hoping to avoid in any viral lung infection. Although it was thought ARDS (acute respiratory distress syndrome) in COVID-19 came from poor lung function accompanied by low oxygen perfusion, it now seems that severe illness and death is caused by blood clots. (See earlier discussion).

If a virus doesn't obey your preventive instruction and ends up hijacking your cells the number one goal changes to guarding against the possibility of pneumonia, particularly a secondary bacterial infection. Often called the silent killer pneumonia can basically suffocate you to death, as may have been the cause of the high mortality of people in 1918 with the deadly cytokine storms. Allopathic doctors make a huge mistake in recommending aspirin or acetaminophen, both absolutely contraindicated in viral infections as noted earlier.

Become familiar with hydrotherapy, botanicals and include essential oils to relieve symptoms. If you have a background in homeopathy apply this modality as well, though now's not the time to take your first case. Maintain hydration. Make sure airways are open and the chest is not feeling constricted. The primary danger in pneumonia is not blood loss but choking.

Be wary of any complications that may lead to pneumonia. Take the temperature because the most common symptoms - cough, shortness of breath, chest pain, headache, muscle aches, fever and chills, fatigue - are also a presentation of almost any viral lung infection. Crackling and wheezing heard on the chest through a stethoscope may lead to a chest x-ray to confirm the presence of fluid.

Pneumonia is particularly deadly for the elderly and young children. Therefore, one cannot overstate the utmost importance of staying on top of healing before the lungs become infected and start filling with fluid.

WHEN TO SEEK HELP

Call your iPCP or go to the hospital any time you are worried and especially having observed any of these symptoms or events:

1. A convulsive fit or you can't wake them up, obviously go to the ER immediately.
2. Lethargy in a child…unresponsive, no eye contact; or inconsolable crying.
3. Meningitis signs: unusual skin rash, severe headache, aversion to light, stiff neck.
4. Difficulty breathing.
5. Any fever lasting longer than 6 hours.
6. Vomiting or diarrhea greater than 24 hours.
7. Fever above 102.2 F in children 3 months to 3 years together with accompanying symptoms.
8. Fever lasting more than 5 days.
9. Body temperature less than 95 F or higher than 103 F or 104 F... this is a tricky one... it depends on the vitality of the person. At least call your doctor.
10. If eyes are glazed or sunken, or there are signs of dehydration.
11. Feeling of confusion or delirium.
12. Any sharp pains anywhere but especially in the right lower abdomen (may be appendix).
13. Blue around the mouth (cyanosis-low oxygen).

For babies add the following:
1. An infant less than three months old with any fever.
2. Convulsions.
3. Listless or the opposite extremely restless.
4. Refuses to be fed.
5. The soft spot on the top of their head is sunken or bulging.
6. A different type of cry or much more than usual.
7. Diarrhea and Vomiting.

> I repeat DO NOT WAIT IF YOU ARE WORRIED. ASK FOR HELP from your integrated primary care provider (iPCP) or GO to the ER.

Do remember, however, to not take or give Acetaminophen[1] or any other fever-reducing drug even though you are scared. This is why you have a well-educated and available PCP. They will give you options.

IF PROCEEDING AT HOME: PURIFY THE SICKROOM

- As a caregiver or patient, wash your hands regularly with diluted herbal essential oils (see below). Do not use toxic substances like Purel®.
- Use a surgical or procedural mask when entering the room to prevent direct transmission of the virus.
- Disinfect surfaces with antimicrobial essential oils like oregano, thyme, peppermint, frankincense, lavender, tea tree, sage, rosemary and lemon. Will reduce transmission of the virus[2].
- Spritz the air with the above aromatherapy oils.
- Change the sheets regularly.
- If there's no fever, make sure to get a little fresh air by opening the windows.
- Let the sunshine or at least light in; this will help with Vitamin D production, cortisol, and aids in disinfecting the room; even during the winter when there is snow and the temperatures are super cold, open the windows for a few minutes periodically to

freshen the room.

TREATMENT: GETTING STARTED TO INITIALLY RELIEVE SUFFERING

Take temperature often...Take the pulse. This is a way to monitor how the patient is...if it changes too slow or too fast. It is also a good way for contact and to soothe.

Have a clipboard so you can write things down easily, as well as what symptoms are predominating, what food they've been given. If things get rough or questionable your iPCP will want to know these things.

1. For Initial Suffering: At the first sign of infection offer a gargle of equal parts crushed garlic, grated ginger and a salt like Himalayan or Hain's Iodized Salt. Add herbs to strengthen the mucosal immunity of the throat. Choose one at a time. (So many to choose from, limiting to these.) Gargle with:
   - Elderberry
   - Licorice
   - Goldenseal (or another berberine-containing herb such as Oregon Grape, Barberry, Goldthread - *Coptis chinensis*
   - Ginger
2. (A) Support for a Cough. If a cough develops water makes the best expectorant but adding herbs - drinking tea - is helpful for mucus thinning, expectoration, and immune support as an added bonus. Choose one or more and have them on hand.
   - Horehound - your grandmother's choice?
   - Cherry bark
   - Elecampane
   - Mullein flowers
   - Slippery Elm Bark
   - Marshmallow Root
   - Helix - Ivy
   - Licorice

   (B) Dry Cough tea recipe. These herbs are mucilages with polysaccharides that expand and become gel-like, protecting irritated tissue. (COVID-19 is known for having a dry cough) For an acute dry cough - (use equal parts of each):

- Mullein flowers
- Coltsfoot leaves
- Marshmallow Root
- Anise Seed (this is also carminative: helps dispels gases from the GI, soothing
- Use 2 teaspoons of dried plant per cup of boiling water, infuse for 20 minutes. Drink this hot several times a day as needed.

3. Inhalation therapy may be helpful at this time. There are a couple of ways to do this:
    - If you have a nebulizer you can use the Neti Pot mixture with a little bit of N-acetyl-cysteine (precursor to glutathione). Inhale for 10-20 minutes two times per day.
    - Another way is to combine Essential Oils (not for children ever and caution with pregnant women) or dry herbs in a pot full of hot water.
    - Cover your head with a towel while leaning over the steam but not too close to get burned and inhale for 10-15 minutes with breaks if needed.
    - Choose Essential Oils from Red Thyme, Rosemary, Peppermint, Cinnamon, Oregano, Clary Sage, Tea Tree.
    - See Botanical and Hydrotherapy chapters for other herbs.
    - If the cough begins to cause tremendous discomfort the infection may have progressed to the point it requires a more serious intervention. Contact your PCP if in any doubt.
4. Diarrhea Support:
    - Carob powder - 2 tsps or more in a bowl of applesauce (always organic, always unsweetened)
5. For Nausea:
    - Ginger tea
6. Quick Energy for exhaustion, confusion, or dizziness:
    - Coconut butter - 1 tbsp. Can add to smoothie or to applesauce.
    - Easy to digest and quickly converted to ketones as the primary fuel source for the brain and muscles.
    - Host of properties, you can substitute it for almond (increased water to grow makes these verboten now) or other nut butters in any recipe.
7. Food:
    - A liquid diet is best: broths, soups, smoothies. (see Recipes)

- See the Optimal Grocery List as in Chapter 13; if a food is in parentheses then it is best to avoid it in the sick room-according to TCM, a cooling food is not desired at this time.
- Also continue suggestions from Chapter 14.
- Give fermented food like sauerkraut, non-dairy yogurt or a probiotic to keep the good gut flora up…if the patient wishes.

8. Homeopathic Support:
   - At the outset *Oscillococcinum*™ is often effective in influenza, although *Aconitum napellus* is also a consideration (often followed by *Gelsemium* or *Belladonna* - what the old homeopathic docs used - see *The People's Home Library* (1910)
   - Or take an original case.
   - Find out the *Genus epidemicus*.
   - For COVID-19 see Homeopathy Chapter.
9. Botanicals:
   - For Influenza use *Lomatium dissectum*, elderberry or licorice.
   - For COVID-19 consider licorice or Ashwaghanda.
10. Hydrotherapy:
    - A wet sheet or wet sock treatment is best done at the outset or if the patient has a strong constitution.
    - In conjunction or otherwise offer cool compresses as needed and give them concoctions that might include lemon juice, raw garlic, and so on from the recipe section.
11. Love:
    - A child needs attention when they are sick. (Well, who doesn't?) As harried and worried as you might be, remember the mind-body connection or psychoneuroimmunology is helped by paying attention to their needs, loving them, even in chaos. This is a chance to be close, to nurture.

BOTTOM LINE

- Convince the patient to rest in bed in a quiet room and to drink plenty of fluids.
- Sip warm broths.
- Add a homeopathic medicine (between eating, as directed) and botanically *lomatium* or another botanical.
- Add phytoplankton or a mushroom or other botanicals (one at a time) to help boost the immune system.

If there is a secondary-infection antibiotics may be considered, otherwise they are useless.

- **CAUTION**: Even if you are feeling confident this still may be a good time to call your health professional to check in and ask for their suggestions.
- If in doubt, make the call.

CHAPTER 16: AFTER THE ILLNESS IS OVER

Any time someone is in intensive care the experience is going to be intense and the recovery may include physical and psychological problems that can take months to years.[1] Especially someone who has been on a mechanical ventilator.

If you are a health professional you may see weakness, dizziness, muscle wasting, disturbance in sleep, severe weight loss, no memory of the event, nightmares, disorientation and other symptoms that must be addressed as these will affect the ability to self-care even in terms of dressing and feeding themselves. There may be depression, anxiety about ever getting well, panic attacks, recurrent and intrusive thoughts; basically PTS, post-traumatic stress. (And remember this may be two to ten years from now. Take a good history.)

The good news is between homeopathic and botanical medicines, eating well with supplementation, keeping well-hydrated, pacing gentle exercise along with still point therapies and meditation can make an enormous difference.

THE PLAN

To rebuild strength and immunity after the event for those who've never been well "since" or after quarantine includes addressing both the physical/physiological,[2] particularly the fatigue (adrenal glands and mitochondria—the powerhouse of our cells), the gut,[3] and any disturbance emotionally whether depression, anxiety, panic attacks, an immobilizing fear of death or another damaging feeling. These must be probed and addressed.

Anyone who tended toward toxic emotions or behaviors before the event will most likely be hampered by previous conditions and beliefs that can put a halt on recovery. An event like COVID-19 has simply shone a light on this. Time to do the emotional work that needs to be done to generate empowered wellness. (Please see my future book, *Transforming Trauma, a drugless and creative path to heal PTSD* for more information and ideas.)

At this time, COVID toes and rashes are a possibility. They last two to three weeks. This could be from medication and the body detoxing and/or from low minerals such as Zinc, Magnesium, Calcium or Vitamins B and C. A multi mineral or phytoplankton may help. Can use calendula cream. If itchy, use baking soda paste or an oat paste. Especially important to hydrate.

FOR YOUR RECOVERY

1. Excellent nutrition: see prevention (* = essential)
   *Superfoods like Phytoplankton (½ tsp/day, depending onproduct, follow directions)
   *Supplements - CoQ-10 400mg, Vitamin C, D, E B complex, Magnesium and other minerals. (see mitochondria support below)
2. Hydration!!!: Alkaline water or water w lemon, teas: Nettles, Dandelion root, Ginger with Turmeric, Green tea (the caffeine may be too stimulating at first).
3. Homeopathics can give the quickest response: *Phosphoricum acidum* (Phosphoric acid) is the most commonly indicated homeopathic medicine when exhaustion continues after the illness has passed. *Scutellaria* may also be considered. A material dose of *Scutellaria* may be warranted for poor sleep. Silica and others can be considered.
4. Botanicals:
   a. *Glycyrrhiza glabra* (licorice) 1/8 tsp three times a day, half (1/16 tsp) for children once to twice a day. (Careful if high blood pressure.)
   b. Ashwagandha 500 mg once a day. Can take more.
   c. An example of a combination is found in Integrative Therapeutics® HPA Adapt - *Rhodiola rosea*, Ashwagandha, Eleuthero, Holy Basil and Maca. Addressing the adrenals and its brain connection is essential.
   d. Mitochondrial support: CoQ-10 and vitamin and mineral recommendations above.

e. Researched Nutritionals® has a great product - ATP 360®. Among other ingredients, PQQ (pyrroloquinoline quinone) an antioxidant that can increase the number of mitochondria), and metabolic helpful substances particularly to restore the lipid membrane.

5. Hydrotherapy: Sauna or daily bath with baking soda, Epsom salts and dead sea salts and essential oils (see chapter). Spritz lavender and roses to boost spirit and increase calm.
6. Be creative: Listen to music that is relaxing. Or play music, sing ...gently, easy. Draw. Write. Everything at your own pace. Pacing: Here is an example of a loved one working through a chronic illness who has been healing the tremendous fatigue. She found pacing and scheduling very helpful and created the following, so she didn't go out of her mind.

09:00AM - 10:00AM	Wake up, eat breakfast
10:00AM - 10:30AM	Stretch gently and review day
10:30AM - 11:00AM	Meditate
11:00AM - 11:30AM	Bounce on ball or trampoline or row for 5 min
11:30AM - 12:30PM	Low/no stimulation rest
12:30PM - 01:00PM	Eat lunch
01:00PM - 01:30PM	Emails, computer, telephone or craft *15-30 min each (mix it up don't spend too long doing any one thing)
01:30PM - 02:30PM	Rest, Read, TV or podcast
02:30PM - 03:00PM	10 min walk and snack
03:00PM - 04:00PM	Rest, Read, TV or podcast
04:00PM - 04:30PM	Emails, computer, telephone or craft *15-30 min each (mix it up don't spend too long doing any one thing)
04:30PM - 05:30PM	Low/no stimulation rest
05:30PM - 06:30PM	Visit with kids play board games
06:30PM - 07:00PM	Eat dinner
07:00PM - 07:30PM	Rest, Read, TV or podcast
07:30PM - 08:00PM	10 min walk (if didn't do walk in afternoon)
08:00PM - 09:00PM	Kids bedtime read
09:00PM - 10:00PM	Bedtime routine meditate and stretching
10:00PM - 11:00PM	Read and go to bed.

Being organized can take the stress out of feeling you're going in circles. You can make an additional chart of what you got done that day whether it's a chore, or project or simply reflecting on what you've learned in terms of healing.

Recovering from a viral infection can take time, especially if your immune system is in a compromised state before the event. This is the reason to get yourself doing all the right things to build up your resistance now.

Continue healing, boosting the mitochondria, adrenals, and your spirits after the acute phase of the viral infection is over, with the tips throughout this book.

A FINAL WORD

My experience since graduating naturopathic medical school in 1987 backs the fact that the combo of preventive measures and non-toxic, antiviral strategies are what is needed to enhance or maintain a robust immune system to counter almost any virus including an epidemic or pandemic.

It is commonly understood that the majority of viruses will mutate to a point that when contracted, symptoms will become milder; however, we must implement lifestyle changes and take appropriate evidence-based medicine to realize this.

A miraculous and multi-level organization, our immune system is well equipped to contain viruses when fed the correct nutrients from foods, plants and supplements as well as having an assured route to detoxify from cellular detritus and/or environmental toxins. And is boosted by homeopathy energetically and psychotherapy emotionally.

Regarding the present novel coronavirus there are more questions than answers in COVID-19 aka SARS-CoV-2 outbreak at this point[1]. It will take at least 18 months to design a vaccine so this is our chance as naturopathic and integrated doctors to show to the extent we can heal novel viruses without resorting to toxic vaccines and as far as possible pharmaceutical drugs.

After the SARS outbreak in 2003, the World Health Organization studied the use of traditional Chinese medicine during that period and determined that they were safe and showed some potential in relieving symptoms such as fatigue and shortness of breath. Jiang Xianfeng, a traditional Chinese medicine practitioner at United Family Health, a top hospital for the affluent in Beijing, added, "Western medicine does not have better answers to this virus. The Chinese people have experienced these sorts of plagues many times in our thousands of years of history. If traditional Chinese medicine was not effective, the Chinese people would already be destroyed."

Researchers from the United States and Taiwan found that certain herbs could suppress the virus if prescribed at specific concentration levels. As we cope with COVID-19, the pandemic that may or may not be the one that we were told was coming, the one benefit is that it is exposing the source of our chronic health disaster that has been our inheritance especially in the United States in 2020.

Perhaps we can learn from Bhutan,[2] the country high in the Himalayas, where there have been 84 confirmed cases of COVID-19 with ZERO deaths! Do you know this is the world's first 100% organic country? Whereas the good ol' USA-we're really not that old at all-where people consume more phosphate per capita than anywhere else in the world, is the hardest hit[3].

Yes, there is definitely a solution to this madness and I pray that this book will help some people avoid the steadily mounting death list.

Did you know that Bhutan is supposed to be one of the kindest nations in the world, its religion[1] being Tibetan Buddhism, led spiritually by the Dalai Lama. So, following the advice of this spiritual leader, above all be gentle and kind with yourself or a loved one during and after sickness, or if you are treating patients. Love and patience will never be squandered in any recovery.

Enjoy the sunrise and sunset and any other parts of nature you can see or feel. Breathe in gratefulness and joy. Go into nature if you can. Forest bathing boosts moods and immune systems.

Thank you for taking care of yourself and all beings.

And remember to check in on your elderly neighbors!

APPENDIX A: RECIPES FOR A STELLAR IMMUNE SYSTEM

This collection of tips and recipes is designed to help your immune system be in tip-top shape, to decrease inflammation, eliminate toxins and provide energy. They do not contain processed foods, high sugar from any source and simple carbohydrates, dairy (except homemade kefir or yogurt from raw milk) or include gluten.

- Use local Farmers Markets and stores that carry fresh, organic produce as much as possible.
- These recipes are perfect for the time of concern when prevention is highest on your list because a virus may be on the horizon, and when you are caring for someone quarantined in the sick room.
- Make sure to know how to make a broth, meat or vegan.
- Honey MUST come from an unpolluted source due to contamination from glyphosate according to Dr. Seneff. Or use another sweetener like stevia or monk fruit.

If you are a busy individual with other responsibilities, think about preparing dishes during the weekend or your days off. Freeze some of the meat and fish dishes with the marinade and thaw them out the night before. They can be put in Pyrex® glass dishes, cover with a lid and freeze.

Tips to keep your immune system in great shape:

- Cook everything from scratch with freshly bought organic foods if possible.
- Cook daily or every other day.
- Do not over or undercook the food.
- Use the least amount of time and heat to cook the food. Some nutrients are best extracted from foods when eaten raw and some when properly cooked (carrots are in this category).
- Keep it simple and tasty.
- If you have family members, cook and prepare food as a family; not only is it more fun but it is beneficial for everyone to learn how healing cooking and food can be.

- Invest in good stainless steel, iron and glass cookware. Cookware is notorious for leaching out metals such as chromium, nickel, aluminum and copper into the food, potentially causing toxicities and allergies.
- As the naturopathic saying goes, "Health begins in the gut." To this end consider adding fermented foods and immune stimulating herbs to favorite recipes. Example: To your favorite non-dairy pesto recipe – add a tbsp. miso and half-teaspoon or so turmeric. You can do the same for any type of stew and stir fries.
- You may use the following recipes in conjunction with the weekly prevention plan in Chapter 13.

DAILY TONIC

MASTER TONIC An Immune Tonic that can be consumed daily by adults			
Ingredients	Apple Cider Vinegar Garlic Ginger Horseradish Root Onion Habanero and Jalapeno Peppers Black Peppercorns Turmeric	Instructions	Blend everything together… room temperature in an air-tight jar for 3 to 4 weeks… Then strained and refrigerated. Take as daily tonic

Alternatively -

- Grapefruit or other juice with ¼ tsp or more of phytoplankton powder.

TEAS: FOR PREVENTION and IN THE SICKROOM

1. Hot water and lemon tea will never go out of style. Lemon is cleansing and alkaline
2. *Cistus incanus:* drink liberally
3. Lemon Balm: antiviral and relaxing, do not take if hypothyroid

4. Peppermint: induces perspiration, cools the body
5. Nettle: cleansing, full of minerals
6. Dandelion: good for liver, full of minerals
7. Ginger Root (rich in healing polysaccharides). Stir and drink 4-6 cups a day...prevention or while sick.
   - Option 1: Grate fresh ginger root and pour boiling water over it. Wait ten minutes. Add ½ tsp turmeric and flax milk. OR
   - Option 2. Cut fresh ginger into slices and cover with water. Slow boil. Can be on the stove all day. OR
   - Option 3. Put 1 pound of fresh ginger root in a blender or Nutribullet® then squeeze out as much as possible to get all of the juice, saving the rest. Add 2 tablespoons of the juice with a bit of lime, dash of cayenne pepper (to taste) to a cup of hot water.

GARLIC GINGER CIDER HONEY (MARY BOVE ND)			
Ingredients	2 cups raw honey (non-polluted source) ½ cup peeled fresh garlic ½ cup grated or sliced fresh ginger root ½ cup cider vinegar	Instructions	Slowly warm honey and vinegar until thin, do not boil. Put ginger and garlic in a wide mouth ball jar. Pour the warmed honey vinegar over it and mix well. Cover. Let stand in warm place for three days shaking daily. Store in the fridge for 3 – 6 months. Use 1-2 teaspoons in hot water or tea

COLD AND FLU TEA (MARY BOVE ND)			
Ingredients	Elder flowers, Linden flowers, Spearmint Herb and Lemon Balm Herb	Instructions	Mix 1 ounce of each in a jar. Use 1- 2 tsp in 8 oz boiling water, steep five minutes covered. Strain and drink hot.

ELDERBERRY TEA			
Ingredients	1 cup fresh elderberries 3 cups water 1 cinnamon stick (optional) 3 whole cloves (optional) 1 teaspoon minced fresh ginger root (optional) 1 cup raw honey (unpolluted source)	Instructions	Place elderberries, water, cinnamon stick, cloves, and ginger in a saucepan over medium heat. Bring to a boil, reduce heat to low, and simmer for 30 minutes. Use a potato masher to mash berries to release juice; strain the mixture through a fine sieve, retaining juice and discarding the pulp. Let juice cool. Stir in honey or stevia until thoroughly combined and transfer to a jar with a lid. Keeps in refrigerator up to 3 months.

JUJUBE TEA - COUGH AND GENERAL IMMUNE BOOSTER
Deborah, a Korean American woman who sells her wares at our farmer's market in Sherman Oaks supplies us with jujubes, also called Red Korean Dates. This fruit, used as a tea, is indicated for flu since it strengthens the immune system and is high in antioxidants. It also aids in emotional balance by decreasing anxiety. • Best combined with ginger and/or licorice as all act synergistically to soothe an achy throat and relieve a cough. • Boil dried or fresh jujubes for hours until concentrated into an extract. • Add ginger and licorice tea as desired. • Sip or swallow small quantities.

GARLIC MAPLE LEMONADE (MARY BOVE ND)			
Ingredients	2 cloves fresh garlic 1 quart of water 1 lemon Maple Syrup (to taste)	Instructions	Finely mince 2 cloves fresh garlic and place in a quart size Mason jar. Fill the jar with boiling water and cover for 30 minutes. Strain out garlic pieces and add the juice of one lemon. Sweeten to taste with maple syrup. Give as warm as possible several times daily.

IMMUNE BOOSTER TEA			
Ingredients	2 sticks Astragalus root 2 Tbsp Dandelion root, roasted 2 Tbsp dried Rosehips 2 Tbsp Nettles 2 Tbsp fresh Ginger, grated 1 tsp Licorice root 1 Cinnamon stick 4 Cloves	Instructions	Add all to 1quart water, simmer covered 20 minutes. Remove from heat and steep another 10 minutes and strain. Add sweetener to taste and stir well. Drink warm 1- 2 times a day.

BREAKFAST RECIPES

Our brains shrink at night so on rising, make sure to always drink a large glass of filtered, alkaline water or fresh lemon squeezed in. Then prepare a quick breakfast that helps decrease inflammation first thing in the morning.

SMOOTHIES

A Nutribullet® is a wonderful contraption! It makes smoothies called Nutriblasts™ that contain all of the fruit and vegetables you need and you can add any supplements as desired. Make sure to use only organic anything. You can also use a VitaMix® machine. Make sure to remove apple seeds, and the pits of cherry, plum, peach and apricots. Do not add ice (stomach muscles will contract). Additions to the vegetables (at least 2/3) and fruits (1/3 max) can be small amounts of:

- Ginger, chia seeds, flax meal, maca root powder, coconut butter, sprouts (broccoli best for detoxing), and even garlic.
- Flax and chia boost omega threes, coconut medium chain fatty acids, and then there are all the minerals, fiber and energy.

At the moment, the addition of kale is controversial because it may concentrate a toxic metal-thallium-from the soil.

BOWL OF NUTS, SEEDS AND BERRIES			
Ingredients	½ cup or more of blueberries or other berries ¼ cup or more of sunflower and pumpkin seeds handful of walnuts 2 tbsp hemp seeds ½ tsp maca powder ¼ tsp cinnamon	Instructions	Add non-dairy milk – flax, coconut, hemp, hazelnut or raw milk (if you know the dairy).

DR. HEATHER'S ANTI-INFLAMMATORY WAKE UP CALL			
Ingredients	2 cups of unsweetened non-dairy milk - can add water to half if desired. 2 scoops pea protein powder 1/16 tsp – ½ tsp phytoplankton (can substitute this for your multi) 1-2 tablespoons hemp seeds 1 tbsp chia seeds or flaxseeds or meal ½ banana (optional) ½ cup to 1 cup fruit preferably blueberries or other berries – can also choose from apples, mangoes, papaya ½ tsp to 1 tsp vitamin C powder or 1 tsp liposomal Vitamin C ½ quercetin powder ½ tsp to 1 tsp maca root powder cinnamon to taste stevia as desired	Instructions	Add to blender or Nutribullet®. Blend. Let sit 15 minutes before drinking. Follow with large glass of filtered, preferably alkaline water. Handful of walnuts and/or almonds, hazelnuts, sunflower seeds if still hungry. Can follow with bromelain and turmeric pills or powder a half hour later for added anti-inflammatory benefits.

LUNCH

There are lunch ideas each day in Dr. Alec's Daily Calender further on. All you really need is a Nutribullet® or Vitamix® filled with vegetables, some fruit, phytoplankton, turmeric and drops of tincture of an adaptogenic herb. Or just have a salad with some protein like garbanzo beans.

BROTHS and SOUPS

Whether you are paleo or vegan, a broth, bone or vegan, may be essential. Know how to make a broth long before the possibility of a sick room stage. Add garlic, onions, leeks, turnips, carrots, parsnips, sweet or purple potatoes, yams, mushrooms especially shitake, maitake, and crimini, enoki.

It can be frozen but make sure to use it within three months. These also come pre-packaged and in powdered form.

Chicken soup or bone broth is gut healing and immune modulating; drinking a cup a day as it is done in many Asian countries for breakfast is a great idea.

Smoothies made with a Nutribullet® or Vitamix® or equivalent (not a blender) can be consumed once or twice a day as they contain all of the fruits and vegetables and will add antioxidants and other essential nutrients with a minimum of fuss.

These can be eaten or sipped any time but it is especially important when someone is sick as they contain an easy and tasty way to get in the minerals needed to heal the body and boost the immune system.

DR ALEC'S BEEF, CHICKEN OR TURKEY STOCK (organically grown only)			
Ingredients	Beef, Chicken or Turkey bones with marrow 2- 3 tbsp Apple cider vinegar 2 bay leaves Black pepper, Himalayan or Celtic salt to taste Vegetables (no nightshade) and herbs to taste	Instructions	Cover beef bones with marrow (or poultry bones) in filtered water in a crockpot. Add about three tablespoons of apple cider vinegar and two to three bay leaves and black pepper and a little bit of Himalayan salt. Add herbs like oregano, marjoram, and thyme for their medicinal value. Turn to low, leave for 2 hours. Then add thinly sliced: Carrots, Onions, Garlic, Broccoli, Cauliflower, Ginger, Mushrooms, any but especially shiitake or reishi. Cook for 30-60 min on high heat until the vegetables are crunchy. 10 min prior to the end of cooking, add thyme, sage, oregano, rosemary and basil to taste.
Everyone is different in what they like. The best thing is to experiment with all of the herbs and vegetables until you find the right combination for your taste. Once you like what you cook, use it weekly to promote health.			

VEGAN BROTH			
Ingredients	A good organic oil - coconut, olive (1 tbsp) Onions, chopped (2 large) Garlic (at least three cloves to as many as you can tolerate) Leeks - white part sliced thinly (2 to 3 medium) Carrots, peeled and chopped (4) Mushrooms (shiitake or reishi) sliced (1 to 2 cups) Bay leaves (2 to 3) Apple cider vinegar (1 tbsp at least) Ginger (½ inch of root or to taste. Powder if root is unavailable.) Herbs to taste. (Oregano, marjoram, basil, thyme, turmeric, curry etc. all have healing properties.)	Instructions	Sauté vegetables in oil, add bay leaves, apple cider vinegar and herbs. Filtered water to cover. Put on low heat for 50 to 60 minutes. You can dilute this with filtered water if it's too strong for you. Add miso only at end - helps by adding beneficial probiotics to the gut.

IMMUNE SUPPORT SOUP (adapted from Mary Bove ND)			
Ingredients	Sauté in 2 tablespoons coconut oil 1 large onion, chopped 3 cloves garlic, minced 1 cup celery, chopped Add: 4 or 5 astragalus sticks 1 cup green beans, chopped, steamed or peas 2 cups carrots or other root veggies – chopped, steamed 1 tsp turmeric 4 cups water with 1 tsp sea salt	Instructions	Combine all in a large pot, simmer gently covered for 30 minutes. Add ¼ cup miso, oregano leaf, both optional and anything that's appropriate for increased antioxidant activity. Add oregano, marjoram, cinnamon, sage, peppermint, thyme, lemon balm - except those with a hypo thyroid.

MISO SOUP
Here is an extremely easy soup that is gut-approved suggested by yoga teacher Claudia MacDonald, Vancouver B.C. Add a teaspoon to a tablespoon (according to taste) of miso paste into hot water. Add scallions or steamed carrots, greens or nothing at all. Sip slowly.

Miscellaneous Recipes

STEAMED VEGETABLES WITH TAMARI GRAVY

(From Dawn Overstreet, Virginia, and my Cape Breton, Nova Scotia neighbor where we were homesteading back in the 1970s!)

Just steaming vegetables is another easy answer, especially if you have a little something healthy as a sauce or marinade to spice them up. The vegetables are better cooked because the heat breaks down the plant's cell wall, releasing nutrients. This can aid absorption.

Sauté ½ small sweet onion diced in a tad bit of coconut oil. Add this to a saucepan of slightly heated 1-½ cups water and ¼ cup Tamari soy sauce or Braggs Liquid Aminos®.

Add 3 tbsps of gluten-free flour. Whisk until smooth with no lumps. Simmer until it becomes thicker.

Add flax or nut milk to thin to your liking.

Add a bit of pepper to taste. Pour it over:

1. Spinach – contains oxalic acid which blocks absorption of iron and calcium and breaks down in high heat. Blanch I minute in boiling water then plunge in ice water before draining.
2. Mushrooms - cooking increases potassium, niacin, zinc and magnesium…all so important for the immune system.
3. Carrots – increases carotenoids like beta-carotenes, precursor to Vitamin A.
4. Asparagus – doubles phenolic acids, a type of polyphenols.
5. Broccoli and Cauliflower - the beneficial enzyme, myrosinase, is released when cooked as well as after chopped if a vegetable is left on a counter for 90 minutes; both can help people with digestive problems to cruciferous vegetables.

IMMUNE NOURISHING BALLS (Mary Bove ND- make sure the kids are building immunity without stressing them.)			
Ingredients	2 tbsp astragalus root powder 1 tsp maca powder 1 tsp each carob and cinnamon powder ½ cup raw honey (unpolluted source) 1 cup tahini or another nut butter	Instructions	Mix well in a large bowl then roll into teaspoon size balls and store in airtight container. Eat 2- 6 balls daily for several weeks.

FERMENTATION FARM'S ORGANIC ELDERBERRY SYRUP			
Ingredients	6 cups water 1 cup organic dried elderberries 1 1/2 cups raw local honey	Instructions	1. In a pot, combine the water and elderberries 2. Bring to a boil and reduce to a simmer for 30 minutes 3. Remove from heat and smash the elderberries to release all remaining juice 4. Strain with a cheesecloth-lined strainer, squeeze then discard the elderberries 5. Let cool to below 100 F then add in the raw honey 6. Mix well using a large whisk 7. Bottle, lid and mark the "made on" date 8. Keep refrigerated, syrup keeps in the fridge for 3-4 weeks
DOSAGE: Adults 1 tbsp 3-4 times per day for relief of flu symptoms and cough Child 1 tsp 3-4 times per day for relief of flu symptoms and cough			

BLACK ELDERBERRY GUMMIES			
Ingredients	1 cup acai juice or another juice, unsweetened 1 tsp agar agar 1 Tbsp raw honey (unpolluted source) 3 oz bottle of elderberry syrup	Instructions	1. Over low heat in a small pan stir together first three ingredients. 2. Heat until agar agar dissolved. 3. Remove from heat and add elderberry syrup. 4. Pour into molds or a glass dish lined with parchment and coated with coconut oil. 5. Freeze for 30 minutes til firm. 6. Pop out of molds or slice. 7. Store on parchment paper inside an airtight container in fridge for up to a week.

Weekly Prevention Plan Recipes

Monday

<table>
<tr><td colspan="4">BREAKFAST
Nut Herb Banana Bread*
This is the time when energy, brain power and stress goes through the roof. There is no time to cook as kids run to school and you must get to work. Use this recipe to prepare everything once a month and freeze the mix in 4 different Pyrex® containers. Thaw one container every Sunday night and bake it for a healthy and filling Monday.</td></tr>
<tr><td>Ingredients</td><td>300g/10½oz/scant 3 cups pecan, hazelnut or walnuts
½ tsp cream of tartar
½ tsp baking soda
1 tsp cinnamon
4 free-range eggs or for vegan
Mix 1 Tbsp flax seeds or meal with 2½ Tbsp water
1 large ripe banana
2 tbsp light olive oil
1 tbsp honey
Fennel, cumin, cardamom seeds
¼ teaspoon of each</td><td>Instructions</td><td>Place the nuts in a grinder or blender and process to form a fine meal.
Place in a bowl with the other dry ingredients.
Place the eggs, banana, oil and honey in a blender and process until smooth.
Pour into the dry ingredients and mix thoroughly.
Spoon into a lined loaf pan. Bake at 180°C/350°F, for 40–45 minutes until firm to touch.
Allow to cool for 5 minutes before turning out.
Slice and serve warm with coconut oil or nut butter.</td></tr>
<tr><td colspan="4">*This can be combined with Dr. Heather's Anti-inflammatory Smoothie.</td></tr>
</table>

JUICE-BASED SMOOTHIE			
Ingredients	1½ cups organic unfiltered apple juice or coconut water or water 2T organic pea or hemp protein powder ½ cup frozen pineapple ½ cup frozen mango 1 banana, sliced ¼ cup of any berries 1 teaspoon of chia, hemp or flax seeds ice as needed	Instructions	Sprinkle of cardamom, cinnamon and nutmeg to taste. Mix all of the ingredients together in a blender; add ice and water for desired consistency. You can add 5 -10 drops of Ashwaganda, Schisandra or Panax ginseng tincture to the smoothie for the added adaptogenic benefit.

LUNCH

Healing Fins

Pick a fish that is on the http://www.seafoodwatch.org/ list that is low on toxicants, high in nutritional value and sustainable. Buy the fish that is recommended for your state. Use this recipe as a guide to cook the fish for a healthy lunch. Marinate in 3 or 4 Pyrex® containers and freeze; thaw desired amount and heat up the night before use, place in fridge, and take to work.

Ingredients	200-400 ml of coconut milk 1 tbsp coconut flour 100ml of vegetable stock or water 2 tsp curry paste ½ tsp ground turmeric 1 garlic clove, crushed 4 fish fillets with or without bones (vegan substitute tempeh or sprouted tofu) 1 red pepper, cut into chunks Handful of cherry tomatoes, halved Sea salt and freshly ground pepper Handful of chopped coriander leaves (cilantro) *Dressing* 1 red grapefruit, peeled 2 clementines or tangerines, peeled 4 oranges, peeled ½ tsp ground cinnamon 1 Tbsp crystallized ginger, chopped Handful of sunflower seeds 2 tbsp of olive oil	Instructions	1. Preheat oven to 180°C/350°F, 2. Mix a little of the coconut milk with the coconut flour to make a paste. Mix into the rest of the coconut milk, vegetable stock, curry paste and spices and pour into a shallow ovenproof dish. 3. Add the fish, red pepper, tomatoes and cook for 20-30 minutes. 4. Season to taste. Sprinkle over the coriander leaves to serve. 5. Combine with a simple green salad* 6. In a separate container make the dressing: cut the grapefruit, clementines and 3 of the oranges into thin slices. Place into a bowl. 7. Juice the remaining orange and olive oil and pour the juice into the bowl with the cinnamon and ginger. 8. Allow to marinate to enhance the flavors. 9. Add to greens just before eating and enjoy a potent antioxidant and detoxing salad bowl. 10. Alternatively, you can buy organic kimchi for the gut support.

*Use any greens that are available to you such as: dark green lettuces include romaine, green leaf, arugula, kale, mustard greens, collard greens, cabbage and broccoli sprouts, dandelion, red clover, plantain, watercress and chickweed. Use about 4 cups for the family of 4 of any combination of the greens that are available.

DINNER

Classic Chicken Soup with Asparagus
(Or beans, lentils, sprouted tofu-cooked separately)

Ingredients	4-6 quarts of broth 2-4 lb of organic chicken 1 onion 4 carrots 4 cloves of garlic Salt and pepper to taste 4 sticks of celery 2 lb of green beans chopped 8 asparagus spears 1 teaspoon of grated ginger 2 Tablespoons of organic soy sauce or Tamari (no wheat) Sauce: soy sauce, 1 clove of crushed garlic and grated ginger	Instructions	You can pre-cut or buy the precut vegetables and keep them in the refrigerator or freezer if they were frozen. Prepare the chicken or vegetable broth as described in the broth section. Keep it frozen in separate containers, so you always have some available. Defrost it when you leave for work in the morning and when you come home put it on the stove right the way for it to start to simmer. Add small pieces of chicken to the broth and cook for about 15-20 minutes, add desired vegetables, and cook for another 20-30 minutes. Alternatively, tofu can be substituted instead of the chicken or separately cooked beans or lentils. Create a mouth-watering ginger soy sauce that you can add to the bowl of soup for a delicious anti-inflammatory and nutritious meal. Combine, add to the bowl of soup to taste and enjoy.

If you like a little bit of carbohydrates, you can always separately cook brown rice, edamame, quinoa, mung beans noodles and eat them with the soup.

SNACKS

The best snacks for Monday combine high antioxidant and energy foods

- Handful of organic nuts or trail mix (no candies)
- Organic gluten and dairy free protein bars
- Handful of blueberries
- A few raw carrots, celeries and broccoli with hummus or a bean dip
- Seeds - Sunflower, hemp, chia, flax
- Nut butters with apples
- Soft boiled egg
- Organic turkey jerky
- Avocado spread and rice crackers
- Cucumbers
- Olives with rice crackers
- Homemade kale chips
- Left over smoothie from morning

Recipe for Energy and Stress Reduction			
Ingredients	Add 1 gram of vitamin C, electrolytes and multivitamin made from a powder or take phytoplankton.	Instructions	Mix well and drink throughout the day. Don't forget to prepare at least 40 ounces of water.

Tuesday

BREAKFAST **Mung Bean Soup** I know it may sound a bit strange but eating soups in the morning is extremely beneficial as they: a) nourish the body with super nutrients and anti-oxidants; b) easy to digest and; c) do not require a lot of time to prepare and eat. Therefore, Tuesday morning requires a calming, high fiber mung bean soup.			
Ingredients	1 cup of sprouted mung beans 1 cup of sprouted black-eye pea beans 1/2 cup of chopped cilantro 4 cloves of garlic Salt to taste Optional: 2 tablespoons of homemade yogurt 1 tablespoon of coconut or olive oil 4 Liters of water or vegetable broth	Instructions	Cook the beans in two separate pots until they are done. Discard the water and wash them again with fresh water in a colander. In a separate large lightly sauté garlic and cilantro in the oil. Add the broth and start simmering. Add the cooked beans.
Mung beans contain high amounts of inositol, which is calming; in addition, they have potent antioxidants, lectins, fiber, protein, magnesium and manganese. All needed for the proper immune function. When combined with black-eye peas, cilantro, garlic and yogurt, the combination provides a potent blend of B vitamins, iron, minerals, healthy fats, and probiotics. And the best thing is that it tastes delicious and is filling. Have a cup of chamomile tea while you are driving to work and enjoy your Tuesday for inflammation control and stress.			

LUNCH

Simple Tuesday Stir-fry

I know it may sound a bit strange but eating soups in the morning is extremely beneficial as they a) nourish the body with super nutrients and anti-oxidants; b) are easy to digest and; c) do not require a lot of time to prepare and eat. Therefore, Tuesday morning requires a calming, high fiber mung bean soup. A good protein is always needed to maintain and repair the body under stress. Dr. Weston Price witnessed numerous times that the endogenous people always preferred organ meats over the muscle meats of the animal as they are most nutrient dense. Animal hearts have the highest amounts of inositol and using them in cooking provides the most nutrient dense foods needed for the intense Tuesday. The following recipe can be used with any kind of protein and is easy to do the day before and eaten for lunch and dinner: (see next page)

Ingredients	1 cup of sprouted mung beans 1 cup of sprouted black-eye pea beans ½ cup of chopped cilantro 4 cloves of garlic Salt to taste Optional: 2 tablespoons of homemade yogurt 1 tablespoon of coconut or olive oil 4 Liters of water or vegetable broth Favorite Vegetables: carrots, broccoli, cauliflower, onions, garlic, celery, asparagus, bok choy, sweet or hot peppers, ginger, green beans, snap peas Asian Sauce: soy sauce, grated ginger and garlic, sesame seeds and oil, anise, red pepper, lime or orange juice. Middle Eastern Sauce: olive or coconut oil, ground turmeric, cumin, saffron, cloves, coriander, cardamom, chili pepper, fennel, lemon grass Western Sauce: olive oil, grated garlic, dried oregano, parsley, basil, rosemary, thyme, sage, and chives	Instructions	Cut any kind of protein into small cubes. You can use chicken or cow's heart, lamb, beef, chicken, or turkey meat. Alternatively, tofu can be used for a great tasting stir-fry. Use any vegetables that you have in your refrigerator (See favorites under ingredients). Cut them into cubes or thinly sliced. Preheat wok and add a little bit of water. It is best to have a stainless steel or iron wok as anodized woks are toxic. Add the meat and cook covered for about 10-20 minutes. Remove the meat and add the vegetables with water and cook for 20-30 minutes. Add the protein to the vegetables and cooked another 10-20 minutes until the meat is done and the vegetables are crunchy. While these ingredients are cooking you can prepare the sauce. There are many ways to make this dish to taste great. Choose your sauce (Asian, Middle Eastern, or Western). Add sauces to the pot 5-10 minutes prior to the end of heating and stir well. Cook brown rice or gluten free noodles in a separate container and combine both into the serving plate for a great nutrient dense and anti-inflammatory dish.
Drink Green Tea with the stir-fry as it contains potent anti-inflammatory and anti-cancer compounds in addition to l-theanine, which is calming.			

DINNER Thyroid Healing Vegetable Salad The second day of the week is gone in a blink of an eye and your body is starting to feel the intensity of the work for the past two days. This calls for the energy, anti-inflammatory, easy to digest and simple dinner that does not require a lot of work. I recommend a thyroid healing vegetable salad.			
Ingredients	Dressing 1 tbsp extra virgin olive or sesame oil 1 tbsp flaxseed oil 1 tbsp rice vinegar 1 tbsp fresh orange or tangerine juice 1 tbsp white miso Salad ½ lb of mixed sea vegetables, such as dulse, arame, nori, sea lettuce and wakame 1-2 lb of green beans cut into 1-inch pieces 1-2 lb of mixed leafy greens Handful of cherry tomatoes, halved Handful of black olives, pitted and halved	Instructions	Mix all the dressing ingredients together while soaking the sea vegetables in water for 5-10 minutes, then drain. Sauté the green beans in boiling water for 5-10 minutes and let them cool off. Combine all the salad ingredients together and drizzle over the dressing. Toss and serve.
It is ok to have some wine with it or sake. Just a tad to help with the relaxation and oxidation. You can always add a little bit of an adaptagenic herb, detoxing and relaxing herbs to it help with the adrenal and immune system recovery. Favorites are oats, lavender, chamomile, passionflower and lavender. Add 5 drops of tincture to the drink and relax for the rest of the night.			

Wednesday

This is the day when the body's energy starting to dip and the inflammation is kicking up a notch. Cooking is the least of your worries and pizza and coffee are becoming your go to. Here are the quickest recipes that can be done in less than 5 minutes but still nutritious and delicious. It is essential to take 5-10-minute breaks throughout the day to just unwind: walk, listen to music, breathing exercises, dance.

BREAKFAST
Prepare the night before. This breakfast is easy to re-heat in the morning and feeds the whole family in 10 minutes before everyone heads out to school or work.
Boil organic eggs for about 5 minutes to make them so the egg yolk is just barely set. Create a quick salad using green leafy vegetables, onions, cooked quinoa (from the night before), avocado and cucumbers. Add olive oil and salt to taste. Cook sweet potato the night before using the following methods: Version A: Take the whole sweet potato, wash it well and remove any strings or damaged parts. Put the whole sweet potato into the Pyrex® baking dish and cook for about 50-70 minutes at 350 F. Version B: cut the potatoes into cubes and add coconut oil with a pinch of cardamom, dry ginger, turmeric, and fennel. Mix and cook in a Pyrex® baking dish for about 50-70 minutes at 350 F. The best way to wash it and let it soak from the morning until night. Wash it again using a sift and put it in the pot with the water just above the quinoa level. Once the quinoa starts to boil remove the foam, turn to simmer, and cook for another 10-15 minutes until no water remains.

LUNCH Again, can be done the night before and warmed up during the day.			
Ingredients	*Non-Starch Options* Broccoli Carrots Brussels sprouts Asparagus Mushrooms	Instructions	Marinate chicken or salmon fillets in any of the sauces described before for the whole day on Sunday and then freeze them inside a Pyrex® baking dish. On Tuesday morning thaw them out in the refrigerator and as soon as you get home, put them in the oven to start cooking. Chicken for about 60 minutes at 350 F, while fish is between 15-20 minutes at 350 degrees. Make a nutritious anti-inflammatory garnish using the vegetables that you have that were already pre-cut from the weekend, night before or frozen. Put them into a steamer or we do not have it, blanch it for 5-10 minutes in hot water. Drain and add any of the sauces you used for the chicken or the fish. While everything is cooking you can squeeze in a 10-15-minute gentle walk for distressing.
Sip on ginger and lemon tea with a bit of honey for digestion and anti-inflammatory properties. Add a store-bought sauerkraut for the added gut healing benefit.			

DINNER Pesto			
Ingredients	1 c basil 4 ½ c olive oil 1-2 TBSP miso A pinch of turmeric Curry Powder 2 Garlic Cloves Salt Pepper	Instructions	Combine in blender with a generous serving of pine nuts; serve over rice noodles, gluten-free pizza, or cooked cauliflower.

Thursday

If you are sick of the cooking for the last three days and just do not have the energy to do it and have the leftovers from the last 2 days, then use them. I always like to make twice as much. Keeping yourself and the family healthy is a full-time job, but it does not have to add to the stress of the everyday life. Again, here are some very quick but nutritious recipes that can be done in the morning and at night in 5 minutes:

BREAKFAST
Soak the oats overnight and cook them in 10 minutes in the morning. Add nuts (brazil nuts are full of selenium), seeds, berries, flaxseed, or chia seeds to the bowl. Have it with a Schizandra tea for the stimulating morning.

LUNCH
Cut up some leftover eggs, add hummus, olives, or marinated artichokes. Mix them all together. Put on gluten free pita or bread and enjoy and simple but delicious sandwich. Combine with a quick Greek salad: Cut cucumbers, tomatoes, avocado and onions. Add olive oil, balsamic vinegar, olives, capers, and salt to taste. Most recipes recommend adding feta but it just not worth it since most are pro-inflammatory.

DINNER
Wash kidney or red beans in a pot of water and soak them starting in the morning. When you come home from work replace the water and start simmering them while removing the white foam. Cook for about 5 minutes and discard the water (this removes some of the phytates that are responsible for the removal of the minerals during the cooking). Replace the water and simmer for another 60 minutes. Drain most of the water and mesh the beans together. Add a little bit of olive oil, crushed garlic, cut onion, salt and spices (chili pepper, cumin, basil, and oregano are my favorites). Cook for another 5-10 minutes. Put on the gluten free taco, add a little bit of a squeezed lemon juice, avocado and enjoy. Two of these will fill you up in a hurry.
DRINK
I love the tacos with a trouble-free detox tomato juice blend. Blend tomatoes, celery, salt, cilantro, basil, mint and parsley, water and a little bit of lemon juice and honey to taste. Chili is another great addition. Drink about 1/2 of a cup as in some people it may irritate the stomach.
CARROT SALAD
Combine with a quick carrot salad that does not need any effort to make. Buy sliced carrots or grate them at home while beans are cooking. Add olive oil, garlic, walnuts, and cranberries. Salt to taste and devour.

Friday

This is it the last day when deadlines are looming and all things imaginable can go wrong. This is the time that requires recipes that reduce the oxidative stress and provide us with the comfort foods, especially at night.

BREAKFAST Simple Antioxidant Shake-
Combine a few peeled oranges, coconut water, Brazil nuts, Vanilla extract, pitted dates, a little bit of lemon juice, Vitamin C, E and a little bit of glutathione and MCT or coconut oil (from your health practitioner). You can also add a little bit of cocoa and protein powder to taste and consistency. Blend them until smooth and enjoy it in the morning and at night on the way back from work.

LUNCH Healthy Butternut Squash Soup Again, you can make this dish the night before and take it to work.
Into a pot add the following: Any kind of cubed squash and cut Broccoli, Celery, Leaks, Fennel, root Carrots, Onion, Garlic, Cauliflower and Asparagus. Add 1/2 of the water usually added to make a soup (about 1/3 of a pot). Cook on low until soft (about 40-60 minutes). Using a hand blender blend everything to a paste consistency. Add ginger, garlic, turmeric, cardamom, fennel, chili peppers and salt to taste. Cook for another 5-10 minutes. Alternatively, you can sauté the vegetables first with spices and coconut oil and then add the water or broth. Enjoy with a gluten free pita or bread and hummus.

DINNER Herb Turkey Burger This is the time when you just want to enjoy your family and have a nice meal that does not drain you any further. This simple but healthy recipe can be used when craving "fast foods".
Combine turkey with finely chopped (in a processor) cilantro, garlic, onion, and parsley. Add ground a little bit of olive oil, cumin, basil, oregano, rosemary, thyme, red or chili peppers and salt to taste. Shape them into patties and put them on a Pyrex® baking dish. Bake at 350 F for about 20-40 minutes. Put it on a gluten free bun with mustard, ketchup, tomato, lettuce, arugula and onion or you can skip the bun and just use lettuce as a wrap. Bake herbed sweet potato fries: Cut a sweet potato into thin slices and add olive oil, rosemary, basil, oregano, and salt. Mix it all together really well to coat the potatoes and bake it in the Pyrex® dish for about 60 min. Make sure it does not burn as this creates carcinogenic acrylamide.
Coleslaw Salad Use this recipe with a simple antioxidant coleslaw salad
Shred a regular green cabbage, red cabbage, and carrots. Create the following antioxidant dressing: Lime juice, honey, apple cider vinegar, olive or sesame oil, ground turmeric and salt. Blend it and mix it with the shredded cabbage. If you crave the mayo - buy and organic one and add it to the blend for a creamier taste.
DESSERT Licorice Cocktail For the desert and a drink, the following great recipes can be used to help to unwind from a busy week and the stress.
Combine 1 part orange juice, 1 part calamansi juice or cooler, 1 part pineapple juice, 1 part cranberry juice. Add honey, vanilla, cinnamon, and nutmeg extract to taste. Add cognac just enough so you can taste the alcohol, but it does not overpower the drink. Add 10 drops of licorice tincture and pour over ice cubes. Shake (do not stir) and enjoy. I do recommend it for kids minus the alcohol. Have it with a small portion of plain dark chocolate or any other chocolate for that matter.

Saturday

This is a relaxation and detoxification day where cooking should be done at minimum and most time spend in meditation, relaxation with minimum food consumption. Light foods should be eaten or water fasting should be done. Use the detoxifying shake recipe from the detoxing section.

Sunday

I recommend using any of the above recipes on Sunday so you can become familiar with them. Involve the whole family and try to brainstorm any of the various combinations together to be healthy and happy.

RECIPES FOR SPECIFIC AILMENTS

SORE THROATS (RECIPE #1)			
Ingredients	2 tbsp raw honey (from unpolluted source) 2 tbsp apple cider vinegar 2 tbsp lemon juice Dash cinnamon	Instructions	Mix well and sip or gargle

SORE THROATS (RECIPE #2)			
Ingredients	Garlic Sea salt Ginger	Instructions	Mix and add to hot water, cover for ten minutes

SORE THROATS (RECIPE #3)			
Ingredients	Onion and Honey (unpolluted source)	Instructions	Cut a whole onion into half. Put in pan and cover with honey Warm the mixture until the onion becomes very soft and you can taste it in the honey. Add chopped garlic for added medicinal benefit. Take 1 tsp 3-4 times a day during sickness. Less if using as prevention (1/2 to 1 tsp.)

FOR ANNOYING MUCUS AND COUCHING
Sip warm flax milk with honey and ginger (can induce sleep).

AN AWESOME DECONGESTANT			
Ingredients	*Part 1* Apple cider vinegar (organic) 1- 4 cups Lemon Juice (organic) -¼ cup *Part 2* a couple of tablespoons raw honey (unpolluted source) ½ to 1 tsp cayenne pepper ½ to 1 tsp grated ginger	Instructions	1. Put part one in a pan and let come to a gentle boil. 2. Take off heat and add part two. 3. Pour into a glass jar. Take two tablespoons daily or one teaspoon for a child.

FOR FEVER
Barley water is an old remedy for high fever when the cause is an infection.

FOR ACHING JOINTS AND MUSCLES
Fenugreek tea with lemon and honey.

FOR SOOTHING SORE THROATS, COUGHS, LARYNGITIS
Make a tea and with these ingredients and sip: • 1 part chopped licorice root • 1 part mullein leaf • 1 part wild cherry bark • add honey (unpolluted source)

FOR COUGHING: THYME HONEY COUGH SYRUP			
Ingredients	1 oz fresh thyme 3 c filtered water ½ c raw honey (unpolluted source)	Instructions	1. Over low heat, add thyme and water to the pan. Put the lid on, though slightly ajar so steam can escape. Simmer on very low until water is reduced to one cup. (Takes a while) 2. Strain off thyme and let cool briefly. 3. Stir in honey. 4. Can store in airtight container in the fridge for up to six weeks. 5. When ill, take 1 teaspoon every few hours to relieve coughing.

FOR DEEP BRONCHIAL COUGHS BRONCHIAL RELAXER FORMULA FROM ROSEMARY GLADSTAR			
Ingredients	1 part licorice root 1 part valerian root ¼ cinnamon bark ¼ part ginger root	Instructions	Prepare an infusion of herbs using 1 to 2 ounces of her herb per quart of water. Let steep for 45 minutes to overnight. Or make a tincture in 80 proof alcohol

FOR SINUS AND CHEST CONGESTION: (SEE HYDROTHERAPY FOR TOPICAL APPLICATION)
For the bath: If you need a change from your standard Epsom salt bath try this: • Peppermint essential oil • Also, tea tree oil and geranium oil.

<table>
<tr><th colspan="4">OLD NATUROPATHIC FORMULA FOR FLU
(John A. Sherman's The Complete Botanical Prescriber, 2nd edition, 1979)</th></tr>
<tr><td>Ingredients</td><td>Achillea (yarrow) – 4 parts
Angelica - 2 parts
Eupatorium perfolatum – 1 part
Mentha pier (mint) – 3 parts
Sambucus (elderberry) – 2 parts</td><td>Instructions</td><td>1. Add 1 ounce to one pint boiling water. Steep.
2. Take ½ cup every 2 – 4 hours</td></tr>
</table>

<table>
<tr><th colspan="4">WARMING CINNAMON BATH
Cinnamon is a warming herb in Chinese medicine. It acts as a decongestant, is antiseptic and can relieve muscle spasms.</th></tr>
<tr><td>Ingredients</td><td>1 cup sea salt (alkaline, and stimulates the release of toxins)
3 tablespoons cinnamon powder</td><td>Instructions</td><td>1. Pour one-quarter of this mixture into a tub full of warm to hot water.
2. Soak for 20-30 minutes.
3. Muscles stiff from acid buildup will relax while the minerals draw out the soreness.</td></tr>
</table>

APPENDIX B: A SOLDIER'S INTAKE IN 1918

TABLE 1: The chart in Table 1 shows a typical soldier's nutritional intake at the time of the Great Flu of 1918

Food	Serving Size	PUFA (g)	Vit A (IU)	Vit C (mg)	Vit D (IU)	Vit E (mg)	Zn (mg)	Se (mcg)	B6 (mg)	B9 (mcg)	B12 (mcg)	Anti-oxidants (mmol/g)[8]
Beef Tenderloin	12 oz	3.3	0	0	0	0	13.3	75.6	0.8	26.4	8.1	31
Bacon	2 oz	2.6	20.8	0	0	0.2	2	34.8	0.2	0.6	0.6	31
Bread	10 oz	0.5	0	0	0	0	3	0	[illegible]	62	0	227
Beans, Canned	3.5 oz	0.2	106	3.1	0	0.2	1.4	4.5	0.1	24	0	69
Rice	1 oz	0	0	0	0	0	0.1	1.6	0	0.3	0	227
Potatoes	16.5 oz	0	15	65	0	0	1.5	0.3	1.5	50	0	303
Carrots	4 oz	0	21383	7.6	0	0.8	0.3	0.1	0.2	24.3	0	303
Tomatoes, Canned	2 oz	0	32.8	2.6	0	0.2	0	0	0	2.2	0	303
Prunes	2 oz	0	986	0	0	0	0.2	0	0.4	1.2	0	278
Banana	1.5 oz	0.1	64.6	8.8	0	0.1	0.2	1	0.4	20.2	0	278
Coffee	1.2 oz	0.1	0	0	0	0	0.1	3.5	0	0	0	2.5
Sugar	5 oz	0	0	0	0	0	0	0	0	0	0	0
Milk, Evaporated	2.5 oz	0	394	1.2	80	0	0.9	2.5	0.[illegible]	9	0.6	0.06
Vinegar	0.3 oz	0	0	0	0	0	0.1	0.2	0	0	0	13.5
Butter	1 oz	0.9	700	0	0	0.6	0	0.3	0	0.8	0	0.06
Cinnamon	0.3 oz	0	7.4	0.1	0	0.1	0	0.1	0	0.1	0	26.5
Total		7.8	24002.2	88.3	80	2.1	24.3	125.4	3.7	224.7	9.3	2100.82

TABLE 2: Recommended Daily Amount for 19 to 30-Year-Old Adults Compared to Soldier's Diet

	PUFA (g)	Vit A (IU)	Vit C (mg)	Vit D (IU)	Vit E (mg)	Zn (mg)	Se (mcg)	B6 (mg)	B9 (mcg)	B12 (mcg)	Anti-oxidants (mmol/g)[8]
Recommended Daily Values	1.6	900	90	600	15	11	55	1.3	400	2.4	Not
Soldier's Daily Totals	7.8	24002.2	88.3	80	2.1	24.3	125.4	3.7	224.7	9.3	2100.82
Net Difference*	6.20	23102.20	-1.70	-520.00	-12.90	13.30	70.40	2.40	-175.30	6.90	N/A

Table 2 calculates the various vitamins and nutrients soldiers received per day as compared to the dietary standard of the normal 19 to 30-Year-Old American male. *A positive net value would indicate an excess in the soldier's daily intake, and a negative value would indicate a deficit.

TABLE 3: Traditional Mediterranean Diet Compared to that of a Soldier in the 1918 Spanish Flu

	PUFA (g)	Vit A (IU)	Vit C (mg)	Vit D (IU)	Vit E (mg)	Zn (mg)	Se (mcg)	B6 (mg)	B9 (mcg)	B12 (mcg)	Anti-oxidants (mmol/g)[8]
Recommended Daily Values	5-11g	1656-	68.8-	16-152	10.1-20.5	8.7-15.8	------	1.14-2.8	189-273	------	Up to 8000[10]
Soldier's Daily Totals	7.8	24002.2	88.3	80	2.1	24.3	125.4	3.7	224.7	9.3	2100.82
Net Difference*	-3.2 to +2.8	+22346.2 to 16599.2	-138.5 to +19.5	-72 to +64	-18.4 to -8	+15.6 to +22.5	N/A	+0.9 to +2.56	-48.3 to +35.7	N/A	-5899.18

*A positive net value would indicate a higher value in American Soldiers, a negative value would intake less in American Soldiers compared to the Mediterranean Diet.

It is worthwhile pointing out that these aforementioned soldiers, on the average, consumed an enormous amount of starchy carbohydrates. Foods with a high glycemic load and index-daily, calculated upwards of 500 grams, the equivalent of 100 teaspoons of white sugar! The booming cigarette industry also contributed to the trench warrior's low immune system by handing out free cigarettes to the troops at every opportunity, known to cause severe damage in the mucosa of the upper and lower respiratory tract. Yet, established medical historians continue to ignore poor nutrition and a compromised immune system as underlying factors behind the Great Flu's deadly assault on the American population.

CONCLUSIONS GATHERED FROM TABLES 1, 2, and 3[1-9]:

In conclusion, we refer to the work of Dr. Weston Price, a heralded nutrition expert and dentist from that era, who, in comparing western and indigenous cultures, concluded the latter's health, including dental, was far superior. Traveling the world, Price came to realize that nutrition in the Western world, from the turn of the century, contained only a fraction of the nutrients consumed by populations who limited themselves to what they could grow, hunt, or catch.

Appendix C: Sources of Toxic Metals and Common Pollutants in Lung Inflammation

Here is a non-inclusive list of what a toxic metal can do to the immune system and how it predisposes us to infection.

TABLE 1: Toxic Metal's Effect on the Body and the Predisposition to Infections[1-9]

Metal	Source	Mechanism of Dysregulation	Organs affected	Exposure routes	Immune system affects
Aluminum	Food, Food Wrapping, Water, Pharmaceuticals, Personal Hygiene Products, Vaccines	Microglia activation - neurotoxicity; Lipid and Protein Oxidation; Mitochondrial Toxin; Disruption of Intestinal Epithelium	Nervous, GI, kidney	Water; Food; Vaccines	Glial and Astrocyte cell activation
Arsenic	Glass and chemical manufacturing, smelters, Fungicides, Pesticides, Herbicides, Animal Feed	Impairs cellular energy production; DNA Hypomethylation	GI tract, nervous system, skin, liver, red blood cells	Air and water; shellfish, chickens	Decreases lymphocyte stimulation, number of macrophages, T regulatory cells
Beryllium	Alloys; Coal Combusion	Development of allergies, corrosive to tissues.	GI tract, respiratory tract (RR); Immune	Air	Lymphocyte proliferation
Cadmium	Electroplating; Galvanizing; Plastic; Paints; Batteries; Parts of Fertilizer; Cigarettes; Welding	Replaces Zn and Ca in enzymes and metabolic systems; Inflammation of the lungs. Blocking of synthesis of vitamin D in kidneys.	GI, RR, kidney, liver, bone, testicle, Immune.	Plants grown on contaminated soil (rice) and animals fed contaminated feed (chicken), water, air.	Increase in pro-inflam. cytokines
Lead	Batteries; Soldering in water pipes; Paint, Electrical Lines	Metabolic systems, glutathione depletion, competes with Ca; Vitamin D metabolism	Nervous, GI, kidney, RBCs	Water; Paint ingestion	Stops macrophages migration; Increase oxidation and stops anti-oxidative properties of neutrophils and macrophages.
Mercury	Fungicide, batteries, dental, fish	Enzyme inhibition, alteration in membrane transport channels, glutathione depletion	Nervous, GI, kidney	Water, seafood,	Toxic to immune cells. Impaired movement to the ingestion of toxin and release of ROS by neutrophils.
Thallium	By product of cadmium, zinc and lead smelter; Coal Power Plants; Electronics; Jewelry	Binds to proteins and enzymes. Replaces potassium; Mitochondrial Toxin	GI tract, kidney, skin	Air; Medical Procedures	None found.
Uranium/Plutonium	Mining and military	Enzyme inhibition; Membrane damage by binding to cellular proteins and phospholipids	GI, kidney, skin	Air; Military wounds	High T cytotoxic and lower T helper cells. Lower number of IgG and IgM antibodies

TABLE 2: Common Pollutants Implicated in Lung Inflammation

	Chemical	Source	Effects	Prevention/Treatment
Indoor Pollutants	Ammonia	Common household cleaners	Irritation of the respiratory tract	Switch to non-toxic cleaners
	Volatile organic compounds: Benzene, Formaldehyde, Xylene, Naphthalene, Styrene, Toluene, Mold, and more	Furnishings, finishes, rug and oven cleaner, paints; Dry cleaning agent; Foam mattress; Cigarette Smoking	Irritants of the respiratory tract; Carcinogenic; Anemia	Removal of the source: Ventilation, Air Purifiers
Outdoor Pollutants	Ozone	Vehicle exhaust; Power plants; Urban Smog	Respiratory irritants; Neurological tissue break down	Stay indoors during poor outdoor air quality; Invest in ai purifiers for the whole home.
	Particulate Matter: PM 10 & PM 2.5	Combustion fuels		
	Sulfur compounds	Coal burning		
	Nitrogen oxide	Combustion fuels		

APPENDIX D: VITAMIN C

A high or at least adequate level of Vitamin C is so important to fight a viral infection.

From the Publisher of Townsend Letter for Doctors October 2014 p 14-15 and reported in many journals since the 1950s, use vitamin C "to palliate, control or eradicate viral infections...other medical alternatives such as ozone, colloidal silver, colostrum, prebiotics, probiotics, proteolytic enzymes, Vitamin D, vitamin A and minerals including magnesium and zinc. As the situation is rapidly worsening and threatening to become an uncontrollable epidemic, it would be reasonable to mandate intravenous vitamin C for all infected individuals as well as health workers treating these patients. Such a mandate would be unprecedented, but urgency calls for unprecedented interventions."

Liposomal Vitamin C (in a lipid base) is said by certain researchers to be as good as intravenous Vitamin C and is able to get into every cell in the body to detox and boost immunity.

HOSPITAL VITAMIN C IV

Dr. Paul Anderson - an article for all you need to know for hospital administration of intravenous Vitamin C.

You can find this article on *International Society for Orthomolecular Medicine's* Website, www.Isom.Ca, under the title *Intravenous Ascorbic Acid for Supportive Treatment in Hospitalized COVID-19 Patients*, published March 24, 2020. Alternatively, you can find it in the journal archives, Volume 35, Number 1, 2020.

CLINIC ANTIVIRAL IV FOR GENERAL IMMUNE SUPPORT

- To be used in a clinic setting. - courtesy of Dr. Clement Lee, NMD, Pasadena, California
- Vit C 5-10g
- 2cc B-complex

- 1cc B6
- 1cc B5
- 3cc Magnesium
- 4cc Calcium
- 2cc Multi Trace Elements (zinc, selenium, manganese, chromium)
- 10cc Lysine
- 1 vial of Engystol® if available

STRONGER IV C DOSAGE

- 25-50g vitamin C
- 3cc Magnesium
- 4cc Calcium
- 3cc Potassium

OZONE IV TREATMENT

- Autohemotherapy with 250cc of blood mixed with 300cc of ozone
  Or
- Ozonated saline of 250-500cc of saline bubbled with ozone for 10 minutes

APPENDIX E: RESOURCES

BOOKS

Perko, Sandra J., *The Homeopathic Treatment of Influenza,* Benchmark Homeopathic Publications, 2005.
Shepard, Dr. Dorothy, *Homeopathy in Epidemic Diseases,* The C.W. Daniel Company Limited, 1967.
Brown, Richard, E., *Rockefeller's Medicine Men,* University of California Press, 1960.
Breslow, Jonathan, *Homeopathic Medicine in the Home,* Ashwins Publications, 1988.
Richardson, Sarah, *Homeopathy - The Illustrated Guide,* Harmony Books, New York, 1989.
Ritter, T. J., *The People's Home Library,* The Imperial Publishing Company, 1919.
Smith, Ed, *Therapeutic Herb Manual,* P.O. Box 116, Williams, Oregon, 1999.
Boericke, William, B., *Organon of Medicine,* Jain Publishers PVT. LTD., 1988.
Moskowitz, Richard, *Vaccines, A Reappraisal,* Skyhorse Publishing, 2017.
Cowan, Thomas, *Vaccines, Autoimmunity,* Chelsea Green Publishing, 2018.
Murray, Michael, Pizzorno, Joseph, *Encyclopedia of Natural Medicine,* Prima Publishing, 1998.
Roberts, Susan, *Naturopathic Pediatric Essentials,* Healing Mountain Publishing Inc., 2003.
Mabey, Richard et al, *The New Age Herbalist,* Collier Books, MacMillan Publishing Company, 1988.
Weiss, Rudolf Fritz, *Herbal Medicine,* Beaconsfield Publishers Ltd., 1988.
Duke, James A., *The Green Pharmacy,* St. Martin's Press, 1997.
Kirchfield, Freidhelm, *Naturopathic Treatment Notebook,* N.C.N.M. Library, 1984.

MY FAVORITE RESOURCES

Local Farmer's Markets - support your local farmer and/or grow your own.

Karen Phytoplankton - pure marine phytoplankton powder (thekarenproject.ca)

Hahnemann Pharmacy - trusted homeopathic medicines. Founded by my beautiful friend, the late Michael Quinn and where I made my first homeopathic medicine, *Bellis perennis*. (hahnemannlabs.com)

Researched Nutritionals - excellent products for detoxification and for mitochondrial support (researchednutritionals.com)

DaVinci Labs - full line of high quality supplements, my source for liposomal Vitamin C (davincilabs.com)

Integrated Therapeutics - my favorite B complex source (active B complex) (integratedtherapeutics.com)

Fermentation Farm - "Healthy Gut = Healthy Life," specializing in probiotic-rich and gut restorative foods dense in nutrients. Located in Orange Co., California (fermfarm.com)

Culture Club - "Improving your microbiome one bite at a time." Pasadena, California (cultureclub101.com)

Barlow Herbal - Home of LDM-100 (*Lomatium dissectum*) via Max Barlow, now run by his daughter Jane. Many potent botanicals. (barlowherbal.com)

Eclectic Institute - wide variety of botanicals, founded by the late naturopathic physician and pharmacist, Ed Alstat, ND. Sandy, Oregon (eclecticherb.com)

Herb Pharm - high quality herbal extracts since 1979 from Ed Smith and Sara Katz (herb-pharm.com)

Wise Woman Herbals - comprehensive source of botanicals (wisewomanherbals.com)

Ayush Herbs – Ayurvedic herbs such as Ashwagandha. Founded by a naturopathic physician (ayush.com)

Mountain Rose Herbs – great selection of organic bulk herbs and spices (mountainroseherbs.com)

Traditional Medicinals – wide range of organic wellness teas (traditionalmedicinals.com)

Jigsaw Health - Magnesium products and other high quality nutritional supplements including Electrolyte Supreme. Scottsdale, AZ (jigsawhealth.com)

Natural Vitality – Magnesium citrate powder, CALM (naturalvitality.com)

Teeccino – Teas, my favorite is their Dandelion Dark Roast with chicory, carob and ramon seeds. Santa Barbara, CA (teeccino.com)

The Body Deli – luxurious organic skin care – Palm Desert, California (thebodydeli.com)

SUGGESTED EQUIPMENT

- Far Infrared Sauna – most economical, can set it up in your bedroom. Removes toxins including plastics and boosts metabolism. (relaxsaunas.com)
- Clearlight Infrared Sauna® – luxurious and elegant (clearlightsaunas.eu)
- Blender – Nutribullet® or Vitamix® or regular blender
- Mini Trampoline - To increase lymph flow 3 – 5 minutes a day.
- Alkaline Water - Enagic Kangen Water® is the Cadillac of alkaline water.

ENDNOTES

Introduction

1. Cara E. We're not ready for the next pandemic. *Gizmodo.* https://gizmodo.com/were-not-ready-for-the-next-pandemic-1839169413. Published October 18, 2019. Accessed October 18, 2019.
2. Cuevas JM, Geller R, Garijo R, López-Aldeguer J, Sanjuán R. Extremely high mutation rate of HIV-1 in vivo. PLoS Biol. 2015;13(9):e1002251. http://dx.doi.org/10.1371/journal.pbio.1002251
3. Arndt W, Mitnik C, Denzler KL, et al. In vitro characterization of a nineteenth-century therapy for smallpox. *PLoS One.* 2012;7(3):e32610. http://dx.doi.org/10.1371/journal.pone.0032610
4. WHO | Vitamin A supplementation. 2015. https://www.who.int/immunization/programmes_systems/interventions/vitamin_A/en/.
5. Zeff JL, Snider P, Myers SP, DeGrandpre Z. The therapeutic order, the determinants of health, and the process of healing in naturopathic medicine and education. in: *The Scientific Basis of Integrative Health.* Taylor & Francis Group, 6000 Broken Sound Parkway NW, Suite 300, Boca Raton, FL 33487-2742: CRC Press; 2017:523-540.
6. Deuster PA, Kemmer CT, Tubbs RDL, Zeno RDS, Minnick MSC, Ac M. The special operations forces nutrition guide. Navyseals.com. https://navyseals.com/wp-content/uploads/2012/12/special-operations-nutrition-guide.pdf. Accessed July 18, 2020. http://dx.doi.org/10.5005/jp/books/10561
7. Osterholm MT. Preparing for the next pandemic. *N Engl J Med.* 2005;352(18):1839-1842.
8. McMurtry, L. Some Can Whistle. *Simon & Schuster,* 2002. Reprint, May 2010.

Chapter One

1. Aiello AE, Larson EL, Sedlak R. Hidden heroes of the health revolution. Sanitation and personal hygiene. *Am J Infect Control.* 2008;36(10 Suppl):S128-51. http://dx.doi.org/10.1016/j.ajic.2008.09.008
2. Kruse H, Kirkemo A-M, Handeland K. Wildlife as source of zoonotic infections. *Emerg Infect Dis.* 2004;10(12):2067-2072.
3. Belongia EA, Naleway AL. Smallpox vaccine: the good, the bad, and the ugly. *Clin Med Res.* 2003;1(2):87-92. http://dx.doi.org/10.3121/cmr.1.2.87
4. Saunders-Hastings PR, Krewski D. Reviewing the history of pandemic influenza: Understanding patterns of emergence and transmission. *Pathogens.* 2016;5(4):66. http://dx.doi.org/10.3390/pathogens5040066
5. Van Epps HL. Influenza: exposing the true killer. *J Exp Med.* 2006;203(4):803. http://dx.doi.org/10.1084/jem.2034fta
6. Youngdahl K. The 1918-19 Spanish Influenza pandemic and vaccine development | history of vaccines. Historyofvaccines.org. https://www.historyofvaccines.org/content/blog/vaccine-development-spanish-flu. Published 2018. Accessed February 3, 2020.

Chapter Two

1. Humphreys M. The influenza of 1918. *Evol Med Public Health.* 2018;2018(1):219-229. http://dx.doi.org/10.1093/emph/eoy024
2. Saunders-Hastings PR, Krewski D. Reviewing the history of pandemic influenza: Understanding patterns of emergence and transmission. *Pathogens.* 2016;5(4):66. http://dx.doi.org/10.3390/pathogens5040066
3. de Vries RP, Peng W, Grant OC, et al. Three mutations switch H7N9 influenza to human-type receptor specificity. *PLoS Pathog.* 2017;13(6):e1006390. http://dx.doi.org/10.1371/journal.ppat.1006390
4. Sun H, Xiao Y, Liu J, et al. Prevalent Eurasian avian-like H1N1

swine influenza virus with 2009 pandemic viral genes facilitating human infection. *Proc Natl Acad Sci U S A*. 2020:201921186. http://dx.doi.org/10.1073/pnas.1921186117

Chapter Three

1. Durbin RK, Kotenko SV, Durbin JE. Interferon induction and function at the mucosal surface. *Immunol Rev*. 2013;255(1):25-39. http://dx.doi.org/10.1111/imr.12101
2. Mackowiak PA. Recycling metchnikoff: probiotics, the intestinal microbiome and the quest for long life. *Front Public Health*. 2013;1:52. http://dx.doi.org/10.3389/fpubh.2013.00052
3. Stoermer KA, Morrison TE. Complement and viral pathogenesis. *Virology*. 2011;411(2):362-373. http://dx.doi.org/10.1016/j.virol.2010.12.045
4. Silwal P, Kim JK, Yuk J-M, Jo E-K. AMP-activated protein kinase and host defense against infection. *Int J Mol Sci*. 2018;19(11):3495 http://dx.doi.org/10.3390/ijms19113495
5. Mao K, Chen S, Chen M, et al. Nitric oxide suppresses NLRP3 inflammasome activation and protects against LPS-induced septic shock. *Cell Res*. 2013;23(2):201-212. http://dx.doi.org/10.1038/cr.2013.6
6. Karunaweera N, Raju R, Gyengesi E, Münch G. Plant polyphenols as inhibitors of NF-ÎoB induced cytokine productionâ€"a potential anti-inflammatory treatment for Alzheimer's disease? *Front Mol Neurosci*. 2015;8:24. http://dx.doi.org/10.3389/fnmol.2015.00024
7. Minodier L, Charrel RN, Ceccaldi P-E, et al. Prevalence of gastrointestinal symptoms in patients with influenza, clinical significance, and pathophysiology of human influenza viruses in faecal samples: what do we know? *Virol J*. 2015;12:215. http://dx.doi.org/10.1186/s12985-015-0448-4
8. Ostaff M, Stange E, Wehkamp J. *Antimicrobial peptides and gut Microbiota in homeostasis and pathology. In: Health and the Gut.* Apple Academic Press; 2014:139-185. http://dx.doi.org/10.1002/emmm.201201773
9. Ye Q, Wang B, Mao J. The pathogenesis and treatment of the `Cytokine Storm' in COVID-19. *J Infect*. 2020;80(6):607-613. http://dx.doi.org/10.1016/j.jinf.2020.03.037

10. Kulkarni AP, Kellaway LA, Kotwal GJ. Herbal complement inhibitors in the treatment of neuroinflammation: future strategy for neuroprotection. *Ann N Y Acad Sci.* 2005;1056(1):413-429.
11. Risitano AM, Mastellos DC, Huber-Lang M, et al. Complement as a target in COVID-19? *Nat Rev Immunol.* 2020;20(6):343-344. http://dx.doi.org/10.1038/s41577-020-0320-7
12. Gralinski LE, Sheahan TP, Morrison TE, et al. Complement activation contributes to severe acute respiratory syndrome Coronavirus pathogenesis. *MBio.* 2018;9(5). http://dx.doi.org/10.1128/mBio.01753-18
13. Endo A, Abbott S, Kucharski AJ, Funk S, Centre for the Mathematical Modelling of Infectious Diseases COVID-19 Working Group. Estimating the overdispersion in COVID-19 transmission using outbreak sizes outside China. *Wellcome Open Res.* 2020;5:67. http://dx.doi.org/10.12688/wellcomeopenres.15842.2
14. Lagishetty V, Liu NQ, Hewison M. Vitamin D metabolism and innate immunity. *Mol Cell Endocrinol.* 2011;347(1-2):97-105. http://dx.doi.org/10.1016/j.mce.2011.04.015
15. Issazadeh-Navikas S, Teimer R, Bockermann R. Influence of dietary components on regulatory T cells. *Mol Med.* 2012;18:95-110. http://dx.doi.org/10.2119/molmed.2011.00311
16. Maggini S, Pierre A, Calder PC. Immune function and micronutrient requirements change over the life course. *Nutrients.* 2018;10(10):1531. http://dx.doi.org/10.3390/nu10101531
17. Statovci D, Aguilera M, MacSharry J, Melgar S. The impact of western diet and nutrients on the Microbiota and immune response at mucosal interfaces. *Front Immunol.* 2017;8:838. http://dx.doi.org/10.3389/fimmu.2017.00838
18. Gawda A, Majka G, Nowak B, Marcinkiewicz J. Air pollution, oxidative stress, and exacerbation of autoimmune diseases. *Cent Eur J Immunol.* 2017;42(3):305-312. http://dx.doi.org/10.5114/ceji.2017.70975
19. Jiang X-Q, Mei X-D, Feng D. Air pollution and chronic airway diseases: what should people know and do? *J Thorac Dis.* 2016;8(1):E31-40. http://dx.doi.org/10.3978/j.issn.2072-1439.2015.11.50
20. Yang Y, Tang H. Aberrant coagulation causes a hyper-

inflammatory response in severe influenza pneumonia. *Cell Mol Immunol*. 2016;13(4):432-442. http://dx.doi.org/10.1038/cmi.2016.1

Chapter Four

1. Schulfer A, Blaser MJ. Risks of antibiotic exposures early in life on the developing microbiome. *PLoS Pathog*. 2015;11(7):e1004903. http://dx.doi.org/10.1371/journal.ppat.1004903
2. Bisanz JE, Enos MK, Mwanga JR, et al. Randomized open-label pilot study of the influence of probiotics and the gut microbiome on toxic metal levels in Tanzanian pregnant women and school children. *MBio*. 2014;5(5):e01580-14. http://dx.doi.org/10.1128/mBio.01580-14
3. Monachese M, Burton JP, Reid G. Bioremediation and tolerance of humans to heavy metals through microbial processes: a potential role for probiotics? *Appl Environ Microbiol*. 2012;78(18):6397-6404. http://dx.doi.org/10.1128/AEM.01665-12
4. Collins S, Reid G. Distant site effects of ingested prebiotics. *Nutrients*. 2016;8(9):523. http://dx.doi.org/10.3390/nu8090523
5. Mackowiak PA. Recycling metchnikoff: probiotics, the intestinal microbiome and the quest for long life. *Front Public Health*. 2013;1:52. http://dx.doi.org/10.3389/fpubh.2013.00052
6. Statovci D, Aguilera M, MacSharry J, Melgar S. The impact of western diet and nutrients on the Microbiota and immune response at mucosal interfaces. *Front Immunol*. 2017;8:838. http://dx.doi.org/10.3389/fimmu.2017.00838
7. Klenner FR. Massive doses of vitamin C and the virus diseases. *South Med Surg*. 1951;113(4):101-107.
8. Schwalfenberg G. Vitamin D for influenza. *Can Fam Physician*. 2015;61(6):507.
9. Razdan K, Singh K, Singh D. Vitamin D Levels and COVID-19 Susceptibility: Is there any Correlation? *Medicine in Drug Discovery*. 2020;7(100051):100051. http://dx.doi.org/10.1016/j.medidd.2020.100051
10. Besedovsky L, Lange T, Born J. Sleep and immune

function. *Pflugers Arch.* 2012;463(1):121-137. http://dx.doi.org/10.1007/s00424-011-1044-0
11. Campos-Rodríguez R, Godínez-Victoria M, Abarca-Rojano E, et al. Stress modulates intestinal secretory immunoglobulin A. *Front Integr Neurosci.* 2013;7:86. http://dx.doi.org/10.3389/fnint.2013.00086
12. Nieman DC, Pedersen BK. Exercise and immune function: Recent developments. *Sports Med.* 1999;27(2):73-80. http://dx.doi.org/10.2165/00007256-199927020-00001
13. Okada, H, Kuhn, C, Feillet, H and Bach, J. The "hygiene hypothesis" for autoimmune and allergic diseases: An update. *Clinical & Experimental Immunology.* 2010;160(1):1-9. http://dx.doi.org/10.1111/j.1365-2249.2010.04139.x
14. Rossi O, van Berkel LA, Chain F, et al. Faecalibacterium prausnitzii A2-165 has a high capacity to induce IL-10 in human and murine dendritic cells and modulates T cell responses. *Sci Rep.* 2016;6(1):18507. http://dx.doi.org/10.1038/srep18507
15. Obata Y, Pachnis V. The effect of Microbiota and the immune system on the development and organization of the Enteric nervous system. *Gastroenterology.* 2016;151(5):836-844. http://dx.doi.org/10.1053/j.gastro.2016.07.044

Chapter Five

1. Kaiser D. In retrospect: The Structure of Scientific Revolutions. *Nature.* 2012;484(7393):164 165. https://doi.org/10.1038/484164a
2. Brown ER. *Rockefeller Medicine Men: Medicine and Capitalism in America.* University of California Press; 1979.
3. Tucker, W.J. *The Gospel of Wealth.* Andover Review VOL XV June 1891, P15.
4. Morgan AL. *Critical Race Theory: A Counternarrative of African American Male Medical Students Attending Predominately White Medical Schools.* 2013.
5. Williams WA, Grandin G. *The Contours of American History.* London, England: Verso Books; 2011.
6. Baïz N, Slama R, Béné M-C, et al. Maternal exposure to air pollution before and during pregnancy related to changes in newborn's cord blood lymphocyte subpopulations. The EDEN

study cohort. *BMC Pregnancy Childbirth*. 2011;11(1):87. http://dx.doi.org/10.1186/1471-2393-11-87
7. Marangoni F, Cetin I, Verduci E, et al. Maternal diet and nutrient requirements in pregnancy and breastfeeding. An Italian consensus document. *Nutrients*. 2016;8(10):629. http://dx.doi.org/10.3390/nu8100629
8. Morrison JL, Regnault TRH. Nutrition in pregnancy: Optimising maternal diet and fetal adaptations to altered nutrient supply. *Nutrients*. 2016;8(6):342. http://dx.doi.org/10.3390/nu8060342
9. Li L, Werler MM. Fruit and vegetable intake and risk of upper respiratory tract infection in pregnant women. *Public Health Nutr*. 2010;13(2):276-282. http://dx.doi.org/10.1017/S1368980009990590.Fruit
10. Geraghty AA, Lindsay KL, Alberdi G, McAuliffe FM, Gibney ER. Nutrition during pregnancy impacts offspring's epigenetic status-evidence from human and animal studies. *Nutr Metab Insights*. 2015;8(Suppl 1):41-47. http://dx.doi.org/10.4137/NMi.s29527.TYPE
11. Clay K, Lewis J, Severnini E. Pollution, infectious disease, and mortality: Evidence from the 1918 Spanish Influenza Pandemic. *J Econ Hist*. 2018;78(04):1179-1209.
12. Armstrong GL, Conn LA, Pinner RW. Trends in infectious disease mortality in the United States during the 20th century. *JAMA*. 1999;281(1):61-66. http://dx.doi.org/10.1001/jama.281.1.61

Chapter Six

1. Hanlon WW. *Pollution and Mortality in the 19th Century*. 2015. http://dx.doi.org/10.3386/w21647
2. Samsel A, Seneff S. Glyphosate, pathways to modern diseases III: Manganese, neurological diseases, and associated pathologies. *Surg Neurol Int*. 2015;6(1):45
3. Genuis SJ, Kelln KL. Toxicant exposure and bioaccumulation: a common and potentially reversible cause of cognitive dysfunction and dementia. *Behav Neurol*. 2015;2015:620143. http://dx.doi.org/10.1155/2015/620143
4. Tintinger GR TAJ. Harmful interactions of non-essential heavy

metals with cells of the innate immune system. *J Clin Toxicol*. 2011;s3(01). http://dx.doi.org/10.4172/2161-0495.s3-005
5. Gies WJ. Some Objections to the Use of Baking Powder. JAMA. 1911;(57):816-821
6. Chey H, Buchanan S. Toxins in everyday life. *Prim Care*. 2008;35(4):707-727. http://dx.doi.org/10.1016/j.pop.2008.07.001
7. Mayer, Jane. *Dark Money: The Hidden History of the Billionaires behind the Rise of the Radical Right*. Anchor Books, Jan 27, 2017.
8. Valavanidis A, Fiotakis K, Vlachogianni T. Airborne particulate matter and human health: toxicological assessment and importance of size and composition of particles for oxidative damage and carcinogenic mechanisms. *J Environ Sci Health C Environ Carcinog Ecotoxicol* Rev. 2008;26(4):339-362. http://dx.doi.org/10.1080/10590500802494538
9. Falcó G, Llobet JM, Bocio A, Domingo JL. Daily intake of arsenic, cadmium, mercury, and lead by consumption of edible marine species. *J Agric Food Chem*. 2006;54(16):6106-6112. http://dx.doi.org/10.1021/jf0610110
10. Anderson RC, Anderson JH. Respiratory toxicity of mattress emissions in mice. *Arch Environ Health*. 2000;55(1):38-43. http://dx.doi.org/10.1080/00039890009603383
11. Mercurio S. *Understanding Toxicology*. Sudbury, MA: Jones and Bartlett; 2016. http://dx.doi.org/10.3390/nu8060342
12. Li L, Werler MM. Fruit and vegetable intake and risk of upper respiratory tract infection in pregnant women. *Public Health Nutr*. 2010;13(2):276-282. http://dx.doi.org/10.1017/S1368980009990590.Fruit
13. Stevens EE, Patrick TE, Pickler R. A history of infant feeding. *J Perinat Educ*. 2009;18(2):32-39. http://dx.doi.org/10.1624/105812409X426314
14. Geraghty AA, Lindsay KL, Alberdi G, McAuliffe FM, Gibney ER. Nutrition during pregnancy impacts offspring's epigenetic status-evidence from human and animal studies. *Nutr Metab Insigh*ts. 2015;8(Suppl 1):41-47. http://dx.doi.org/10.4137/NMi.s29527.TYPE
15. Landrigan PJ, Goldman LR. Children's vulnerability to toxic chemicals: a challenge and opportunity to strengthen health and environmental policy. *Health Aff (Millwood)*. 2011;30(5):842-850. http://dx.doi.org/10.1377/hlthaff.2011.0151
16. Bruckner JV. Differences in sensitivity of children and adults to

chemical toxicity: the NAS panel report. *Regul Toxicol Pharmacol.* 2000;31(3):280-285. http://dx.doi.org/10.1006/rtph.2000.1393
17. Scheuplein R, Charnley G, Dourson M. Differential sensitivity of children and adults to chemical toxicity. I. Biological basis. *Regul Toxicol Pharmacol.* 2002;35(3):429-447. http://dx.doi.org/10.1006/rtph.2002.1558
18. Gross R. Beyond food and nutrition: How can cities be made healthy? *Asia Pac J Clin Nutr.* 2002;11(s9):S763-S766.
19. Seneff S, Davidson RM, Lauritzen A, Samsel A, Wainwright G. A novel hypothesis for atherosclerosis as a cholesterol sulfate deficiency syndrome. *Theor Biol Med Model.* 2015;12(1):9. http://dx.doi.org/10.1186/s12976-015-0006-1
20. Samsel A, Seneff S. Glyphosate's suppression of cytochrome P450 enzymes and amino acid biosynthesis by the gut microbiome: Pathways to modern diseases. *Entropy (Basel).* 2013;15(12):1416-1463. http://dx.doi.org/10.4103/2152-7806.153876
21. Lane J. Aviation biofuels: which airlines are doing what, with whom? Biofuelsdigest.com. https://www.biofuelsdigest.com/bdigest/2012/06/05/aviation-biofuels-which-airlines-are-doing-what-with-whom/.
22. FDA.gov.
23. Schofield K. The metal neurotoxins: An important role in current human neural epidemics? Int J *Environ Res Public Health.* 2017;14(12). http://dx.doi.org/10.3390/ijerph14121511
24. Watad A, David P, Brown S, Shoenfeld Y. Autoimmune/inflammatory syndrome induced by adjuvants and thyroid autoimmunity. *Front Endocrinol (Lausanne).* 2016;7:150. http://dx.doi.org/10.3389/fendo.2016.00150
25. Cowan T. *Vaccines, Autoimmunity, and the Changing Nature of Childhood Illness.* White River Junction, VT: Chelsea Green Publishing; 2018.
26. Buttram HE. Current childhood vaccine programs: An overview with emphasis on the Measles-Mumps-Rubella (MMR) vaccine and of its compromising of the mucosal immune system. *HE Buttram/Medi cal Veritas.* 2008;5:1820-1827. http://dx.doi.org/10.1588/medver/2008.05.00190

Chapter Seven

1. Gold JAW, Wong KK, Szablewski CM, et al. Characteristics and clinical outcomes of adult patients hospitalized with COVID-19 - Georgia, March 2020. *MMWR Morb Mortal Wkly Rep.* 2020;69(18):545-550. http://dx.doi.org/10.15585/mmwr.mm6918e1external icon
2. Guan W et al. Co-morbidity and its impact on 1590 patients with COVID-19 in China: a nationwide analysis. *European Respiratory Journal* 2020 55: 2000547; DOI: 10.1183/13993003.00547-2020
3. Wang K, Chen W, Zhou Y-S, et al. SARS-CoV-2 invades host cells via a novel route: CD147-spike protein. *bioRxiv.* 2020. http://dx.doi.org/10.1101/2020.03.14.988345
4. CDC COVID-19 Response Team. Preliminary estimates of the prevalence of selected underlying health conditions among patients with Coronavirus Disease 2019 - United States, February 12-March 28, 2020. *MMWR Morb Mortal Wkly Rep.* 2020;69(13):382-386. http://dx.doi.org/10.15585/mmwr.mm6913e2external icon
5. CDC.org. June 25, 2020.
6. Loh D. The potential of melatonin in the prevention and attenuation of oxidative hemolysis and myocardial injury from cd147 SARS-CoV-2 spike protein receptor binding. *Melatonin Res.* 2020;3(3):380-416. http://dx.doi.org/10.32794/mr11250069
7. Tahamtan A, Ardebili A. Real-time RT-PCR in COVID-19 detection: issues affecting the results. *Expert Rev Mol Diagn.* 2020;20(5):453-454. http://dx.doi.org/10.1080/14737159.2020.1757437
8. Davies G, Garami AR, Byers JC. Evidence supports a causal role for vitamin D status in COVID-19 outcomes. *bioRxiv.* 2020. http://dx.doi.org/10.1101/2020.05.01.20087965
9. Gerlach H. Agents to reduce cytokine storm. *F1000Res.* 2016;5:2909. http://dx.doi.org/10.12688/f1000research.9092.1
10. Kumar A, Kubota Y, Chernov M, Kasuya H. Potential role of zinc supplementation in prophylaxis and treatment of COVID-19. *Med Hypotheses.* 2020;144(109848):109848. http://dx.doi.org/10.1016/j.mehy.2020.109848
11. Boretti A, Banik BK. Intravenous Vitamin C for reduction of cytokines storm in Acute Respiratory Distress Syndrome. *PharmaNutrition.* 2020;12(100190):100190.

http://dx.doi.org/10.1016/j.phanu.2020.100190

12. Polonikov A. Endogenous deficiency of glutathione as the most likely cause of serious manifestations and death in COVID-19 patients. *ACS Infect Dis*. 2020;6(7):1558-1562. http://dx.doi.org/10.1021/acsinfecdis.0c00288
13. Roshanravan N, Ghaffari S, Hedayati M. Angiotensin converting enzyme-2 as therapeutic target in COVID-19. *Diabetes Metab Syndr*. 2020;14(4):637-639. http://dx.doi.org/10.1016/j.dsx.2020.05.0226
14. Wu C, Zheng S, Chen Y, Zheng M. Single-cell RNA expression profiling of ACE2, the putative receptor of Wuhan 2019-nCoV, in the nasal tissue. *bioRxiv*. 2020. doi:10.1101/2020.02.11.20022228. http://dx.doi.org/10.1101/2020.01.26.919985
15. Mao K, Chen S, Chen M, et al. Nitric oxide suppresses NLRP3 inflammasome activation and protects against LPS-induced septic shock. *Cell Res*. 2013;23(2):201-212. http://dx.doi.org/10.1038/cr.2013.6
16. Magro C, Mulvey JJ, Berlin D, et al. Complement associated microvascular injury and thrombosis in the pathogenesis of severe COVID-19 infection: A report of five cases. *Transl Res*. 2020;220:1-13. http://dx.doi.org/10.1016/j.trsl.2020.04.007
17. Wenzhong L, Hualan L. COVID-19: Attacks the 1-beta chain of hemoglobin and captures the porphyrin to inhibit human heme metabolism. *ChemRxiv*. 2020. http://dx.doi.org/10.26434/chemrxiv.11938173.v7
18. Wu H-M, Zhao C-C, Xie Q-M, Xu J, Fei G-H. TLR2-melatonin feedback loop regulates the activation of NLRP3 inflammasome in Murine allergic airway inflammation. *Front Immunol*. 2020;11:172. http://dx.doi.org/10.3389/fimmu.2020.00172
19. Kung C-M, Tseng Z-L, Wang H-L. Erythrocyte fragility increases with level of glycosylated hemoglobin in type 2 diabetic patients. *Clin Hemorheol Microcirc*. 2009;43(4):345-351. http://dx.doi.org/10.3233/CH-2009-1245
20. Zhang R, Wang X, Ni L, et al. COVID-19: Melatonin as a potential adjuvant treatment. *Life Sci*. 2020;250(117583):117583. http://dx.doi.org/10.1016/j.lfs.2020.117583
21. Zhang Y, Li X, Grailer JJ, et al. Melatonin alleviates acute lung injury through inhibiting the NLRP3 inflammasome. *J Pineal Res*. 2016;60(4):405-414. http://dx.doi.org/10.1111/jpi.12322

22. Wink DA, Hines HB, Cheng RYS, et al. Nitric oxide and redox mechanisms in the immune response. *J Leukoc Biol.* 2011;89(6):873-891. http://dx.doi.org/10.1189/jlb.1010550
23. Sureda A, Batle JM, Tauler P, Ferrer MD, Tur JA, Pons A. Vitamin C supplementation influences the antioxidant response and nitric oxide handling of erythrocytes and lymphocytes to diving apnea. *Eur J Clin Nutr.* 2006;60(7):838-846. http://dx.doi.org/10.1038/sj.ejcn.1602388
24. Yurchenko V, Constant S, Eisenmesser E, Bukrinsky M. Cyclophilin-CD147 interactions: a new target for anti-inflammatory therapeutics: CD147-cyclophilin interactions. *Clin Exp Immunol.* 2010;160(3):305-317.
25. Fox SE, Akmatbekov A, Harbert JL, Li G, Quincy Brown J, Vander Heide RS. Pulmonary and cardiac pathology in African American patients with COVID-19: an autopsy series from New Orleans. *Lancet Respir Med.* 2020;8(7):681-686. http://dx.doi.org/10.1016/S2213-2600(20)30243-5

Chapter Eight

1. Jacobs J. Homeopathic prevention and management of epidemic diseases. *Homeopathy.* 2018;107(3):157-160. http://dx.doi.org/10.1055/s-0038-1649487
2. Morrell P. *Hahnemann's Homoeopathy.* New Delhi, India: B Jain; 2004.
3. Jacobs J, Guthrie BL, Montes GA, et al. Homeopathic combination remedy in the treatment of acute childhood diarrhea in Honduras. *J Altern Complement Med.* 2006;12(8):723-732. http://dx.doi.org/10.1089/acm.2006.12.723
4. Tessier JP. *Recherches Cliniques Sur Le Traitement De La Pneumonie Et Du Choléra Suivant La Méthode De Hahnemann: Précédées D'une Introduction Sur L'abus De La Statistique En Médecine.* France: Nabu Press; 2012.
5. Photothéque Homéopathique présentée par Homéopathe International. Homeoint.org. http://www.homeoint.org/photo/.
6. Shepperd J. Hahnemann's pure method of science. Centerforintegralhealth.com. https://centerforintegralhealth.com/wp-

content/uploads/2019/10/Shepperd_Simillimum_2002__Hahnemanns_Pure_Method_of_Science.pdf. Published 2002.
7. Smith CB. *Champion of Homoeopathy: Life of Dr. Margery Blackie.* London, England: John Murray; 1986; 38.
8. How to cure influenza - Ethelbert Petrie Hoyle. Hpathy.com. https://hpathy.com/homeopathy-papers/cure-influenza/.
9. Anastopoulos C. *Particle or Wave: The Evolution of the Concept of Matter in Modern Physics.* Princeton, NJ: Princeton University Press; 2008.
10. Saine A. JAHC2020 Online Global Summit. Dr Heather Uncensored
11. Samet L. JAHC2020 Online Global Summit. Dr Heather Uncensored
12. Milgrom LR. Patient-practitioner-remedy (PPR) entanglement. Part 2: Extending the metaphor for homeopathy using molecular quantum theory. *Homeopathy.* 2003;92(1):35-43.
13. Dean M. Comparative evaluation of homeopathy and allopathy within the Parisian hospital system, 1849-1851. *J R Soc Med.* 2010;103(1):34-36.

Chapter Nine

1. Wee S-L. In Coronavirus, China weighs benefits of buffalo horn and other remedies. The New York times. https://www.nytimes.com/2020/02/05/world/asia/coronavirus-traditional-chinese-medicine.html. Published February 5, 2020. Accessed January 5, 2020.
2. Ren Y, Qiao W, Fu D, et al. Traditional Chinese medicine protects against cytokine production as the potential immunosuppressive agents in atherosclerosis. *J Immunol Res.* 2017;2017:7424307. http://dx.doi.org/10.1155/2017/7424307
3. Tian L, Wang Z, Wu H, et al. Evaluation of the anti-neuraminidase activity of the traditional Chinese medicines and determination of the anti-influenza A virus effects of the neuraminidase inhibitory TCMs in vitro and in vivo. *J Ethnopharmacol.* 2011;137(1):534-542. http://dx.doi.org/10.1016/j.jep.2011.06.002
4. Yin M, Zhang Y, Li H. Advances in research on immunoregulation of macrophages by plant

polysaccharides. *Front Immunol.* 2019;10:145. http://dx.doi.org/10.3389/fimmu.2019.00145
5. Iguchi M, Littmann AE, Chang S-H, Wester LA, Knipper JS, Shields RK. Heat stress and cardiovascular, hormonal, and heat shock proteins in humans. *J Athl Train.* 2012;47(2):184-190.
6. Alleva LM, Cai C, Clark IA. Using complementary and alternative medicines to target the host response during severe influenza. *Evid Based Complement Alternat Med.* 2010;7(4):501-510. http://dx.doi.org/10.1093/ecam/nep152
7. Prasad A, Muthamilarasan M, Prasad M. Synergistic antiviral effects against SARS-CoV-2 by plant-based molecules [published online ahead of print, 2020 Jun 19]. *Plant Cell Rep.* 2020;1-6. doi:10.1007/s00299-020-02560-w
8. Utsunomiya H, Ichinose M, Ikeda K, et al. Inhibition by caffeic acid of the influenza A virus multiplication in vitro. *Int J Mol Med.* 2014;34(4):1020-1024. http://dx.doi.org/10.3892/ijmm.2014.1859
9. Kuang Y, Li B, Fan J, Qiao X, Ye M. Antitussive and expectorant activities of licorice and its major compounds. *Bioorg Med Chem.* 2018;26(1):278-284. http://dx.doi.org/10.1016/j.bmc.2017.11.046
10. Yang Y, Islam MS, Wang J, Li Y, Chen X. Traditional Chinese Medicine in the treatment of patients infected with 2019-new Coronavirus (SARS-CoV-2): A review and perspective. *Int J Biol Sci.* 2020;16(10):1708-1717. http://dx.doi.org/10.7150/ijbs.45538
11. McCutcheon AR, Roberts TE, Gibbons E, et al. Antiviral screening of British Columbian medicinal plants. *J Ethnopharmacol.* 1995;49(2):101-110.
12. Weng j-R. "Antiviral activity of Sambucus Formoosana Nakai." *Virus Res* Vol 273, Nov 2019, 197767 https://doi.org/10.1016/j.virusres.2019.197767
13. Shamaki U, Abdul-Dahiru E-Y, Abdulrahman I, Ogbe O. In vitro inhibition of neuraminidase activity of influenza virus (H5N2) by methanolic soluble fraction of Ganoderma lucidum extract. Modernscientificpress.com. http://www.modernscientificpress.com/Journals/downloadFile.aspx?oNi57mI9FIF9OKRLCcg8Ec3yGvEOALf8gTIsFW/oOOCahPHTboXd/wzixXRXoc8t.
14. Cinatl J, Morgenstern B, Bauer G, Chandra P, Rabenau H, Doerr HW. Glycyrrhizin, an active component of liquorice roots, and replication of SARS-associated coronavirus. *Lancet.*

2003;361(9374):2045-2046.
15. Mukhtar M, Arshad M, Ahmad M, Pomerantz RJ, Wigdahl B, Parveen Z. Antiviral potentials of medicinal plants. *Virus Res.* 2008;131(2):111-120. http://dx.doi.org/10.1016/j.virusres.2007.09.008
16. Barlow, J. In conversation on podcast Dr. Heather Uncensored, Episode 2.
17. Barak V, Halperin T, Kalickman I. The effect of Sambucol, a black elderberry-based, natural product, on the production of human cytokines: I. Inflammatory cytokines. *Eur Cytokine Netw.* 2001;12(2):290-296.
18. Utsunomiya T, Kobayashi M, Pollard RB, Suzuki F. Glycyrrhizin, an active component of licorice roots, reduces morbidity and mortality of mice infected with lethal doses of influenza virus. *Antimicrob Agents Chemother.* 1997;41(3):551-556.
19. Kumar V, Dhanjal JK, Kaul SC, Wadhwa R, Sundar D. Withanone and caffeic acid phenethyl ester are predicted to interact with main protease (Mpro) of SARS-CoV-2 and inhibit its activity. *J Biomol Struct Dyn.* 2020:1-13. http://dx.doi.org/10.1080/07391102.2020.1772108
20. Cai Z, Zhang G, Tang B, Liu Y, Fu X, Zhang X. Promising anti-influenza properties of active constituent of Withania somnifera ayurvedic herb in targeting neuraminidase of H1N1 influenza: Computational study. *Cell Biochem Biophys.* 2015;72(3):727-739. http://dx.doi.org/10.1007/s12013-015-0524-9
21. Puri HS. Rasayana: Ayurvedic herbs for longevity and rejuvenation: Volume 2 of traditional herbal medicines for modern times. *J Altern Complement Med.* 2003;9(2):331-332.
22. Williamson EM. *Major Herbs of Ayurveda.* London, England: Churchill Livingstone; 2002.
23. Kapoor LD. *CRC Handbook of Ayurvedic Medicinal Plants*: Boca Raton, FL. CRC Press; 1990.
24. Monograph. Withania somnifera. *Altern Med Rev.* 2004;9(2):211-214.
25. Singh N, Bhalla M, De Jager P, Gilca M. An Overview on Ashwagandha: A Rasayana (Rejuvenator) of Ayurveda. *Afr J Tradit Complement Altern Med.* 2011;8(5S). http://dx.doi.org/10.4314/ajtcam.v8i5ss.9
26. Nayak MK, Agrawal AS, Bose S, et al. Antiviral activity of baicalin against influenza virus H1N1-pdm09 is due to

modulation of NS1-mediated cellular innate immune responses. *J Antimicrob Chemother*. 2014;69(5):1298-1310. http://dx.doi.org/10.1093/jac/dkt534

27. Hour M-J, Huang S-H, Chang C-Y, et al. Baicalein, ethyl acetate, and chloroform extracts of Scutellaria baicalensis inhibit the neuraminidase activity of pandemic 2009 H1N1 and seasonal influenza A viruses. *Evid Based Complement Alternat Med*. 2013;2013:750803. http://dx.doi.org/10.1155/2013/750803
28. Holzinger F, Chenot J-F. Systematic review of clinical trials assessing the effectiveness of ivy leaf (hedera helix) for acute upper respiratory tract infections. *Evid Based Complement Alternat Med*. 2011;2011:382789. http://dx.doi.org/10.1155/2011/382789
29. Guan W et al. Co-morbidity and its impact on 1590 patients with COVID-19 in China: a nationwide analysis. *European Respiratory Journal* 2020 55: 2000547; DOI: 10.1183/13993003.00547-2020
30. Quan FS, Compans RW, Cho Y-K, Kang S-M. Ginseng and Salviae herbs play a role as immune activators and modulate immune responses during influenza virus infection. *Vacci ne*. 2007;25(2):272-282. http://dx.doi.org/10.1016/j.vaccine.2006.07.041

Chapter Ten

1. Crinnion WJ. Sauna as a valuable clinical tool for cardiovascular, autoimmune, toxicant- induced and other chronic health problems. *Altern Med Rev*. 2011;16(3):215-225.
2. Grüber C, Riesberg A, Mansmann U, Knipschild P, Wahn U, Bühring M. The effect of hydrotherapy on the incidence of common cold episodes in children: a randomised clinical trial. *Eur J Pediatr*. 2003;162(3):168-176. http://dx.doi.org/10.1007/s00431-002-1138-y
3. Pilch W, Pokora I, Szygu□a Z, et al. Effect of a single finnish sauna session on white blood cell profile and cortisol levels in athletes and non-athletes. *J Hum Kinet*. 2013;39(1):127-135. http://dx.doi.org/10.2478/hukin-2013-0075
4. Huyck A, Broderick K. Hydrotherapy. In: Textbook of Natural Medicine. *Elsevier;* 2013:327-337. http://dx.doi.org/10.1016/B978-1-4377-2333-5.00040-7

5. Pourghanbari G, Nili H, Moattari A, Mohammadi A, Iraji A. Antiviral activity of the oseltamivir and Melissa officinalis L. essential oil against avian influenza A virus (H9N2). *Virusdisease*. 2016;27(2):170-178. doi:10.1007/s13337-016-0321-0
6. Choi H-J. Chemical constituents of essential oils possessing anti-influenza A/WS/33 virus activity. *Osong Public Health Res Perspect*. 2018;9(6):348-353. http://dx.doi.org/10.24171/j.phrp.2018.9.6.09
7. Ma L, Yao L. Antiviral Effects of Plant-Derived Essential Oils and Their Components: An Updated Review. *Molecules*. 2020; 25(11):2627. Published 2020 Jun 5. doi:10.3390/molecules25112627

Chapter Eleven

1. Neustadt J. Western Diet and Inflammation. Integr Med. 2006;5(4):14-18.
2. Sanchez A, Reeser JL, Lau HS, et al. Role of sugars in human neutrophilic phagocytosis. *Am J Clin Nutr*. 1973;26(11):1180-1184.
3. Ilyas R, Wallis R, Soilleux EJ, et al. High glucose disrupts oligosaccharide recognition function via competitive inhibition: a potential mechanism for immune dysregulation in diabetes mellitus. *Immunobiology*. 2011;216(1-2):126-131. http://dx.doi.org/10.1016/j.imbio.2010.06.002
4. Davidson NJ, Sowden JM, Fletcher J. Defective phagocytosis in insulin controlled diabetics: evidence for a reaction between glucose and opsonising proteins. *J Clin Pathol*. 1984;37(7):783-786. http://dx.doi.org/10.1136/jcp.37.7.783
5. Lagarda-Diaz I, Guzman-Partida AM, Vazquez-Moreno L. Legume lectins: Proteins with diverse applications. *Int J Mol Sci*. 2017;18(6). http://dx.doi.org/10.3390/ijms18061242
6. Mason CP, Tarr AW. Human lectins and their roles in viral infections. *Molecules*. 2015;20(2):2229-2271. http://dx.doi.org/10.3390/molecules20022229
7. Jiang Y, Yang G, Wang Q, et al. Molecular mechanisms underlying protection against H9N2 influenza virus challenge in mice by recombinant Lactobacillus plantarum with surface

displayed HA2-LTB. *J Biotechnol.* 2017;259:6-14.
8. Utsunomiya H, Ichinose M, Ikeda K, et al. Inhibition by caffeic acid of the influenza A virus multiplication in vitro. *Int J Mol Med.* 2014;34(4):1020-1024. http://dx.doi.org/10.3892/ijmm.2014.1859
9. Holmström KM, Kostov RV, Dinkova-Kostova AT. The multifaceted role of Nrf2 in mitochondrial function. *Curr Opin Toxicol.* 2016;1:80-91. http://dx.doi.org/10.1016/j.cotox.2016.10.002
10. Van Duyn MA, Pivonka E. Overview of the health benefits of fruit and vegetable consumption for the dietetics professional: selected literature. *J Am Diet Assoc.* 2000;100(12):1511-1521. http://dx.doi.org/10.1089/fpd.2009.0477
11. T□zsér J. and Benk□ S. Natural Compounds as Regulators of NLRP3 Inflammasome-Mediated IL-1□ Production. *Mediators of Inflammation.* Volume 2016 (2016), Review article ID 5460302, http://dx.doi.org/10.1155/2016/5460302
12. Molfino A, Gioia G, Rossi Fanelli F, Muscaritoli M. The role for dietary omega-3 fatty acids supplementation in older adults. *Nutrients.* 2014;6(10):4058-4073. Published 2014 Oct 3. doi:10.3390/nu6104058
13. Shoenfeld Y, Azrielant S. Vitamin D and autoimmune diseases. *Indian j rheumatol.* 2017;12(4):219. http://dx.doi.org/10.4103/injr.injr
14. Mawson AR. Role of fat-soluble vitamins A and D in the pathogenesis of influenza: A new perspective. *ISRN Infect Dis.* 2013; 2013:1-26. http://dx.doi.org/10.5402/2013/246737
15. McFarlin BK, Carpenter KC, Davidson T, McFarlin MA. Baker's yeast beta glucan supplementation increases salivary IgA and decreases cold/flu symptomatic days after intense exercise. *J Diet Suppl.* 2013;10(3):171-183. http://dx.doi.org/10.3109/19390211.2013.820248
16. Bashir KMI, Choi J-S. Clinical and physiological perspectives of □-glucans: The past, present, and future. *Int J Mol Sci.* 2017;18(9). http://dx.doi.org/10.3390/ijms18091906
17. Cesarone MR, Belcaro G, Di Renzo A, et al. Prevention of influenza episodes with colostrum compared with vaccination in healthy and high-risk cardiovascular subjects: the epidemiologic study in San Valentino: The epidemiologic study in San Valentino. *Clin Appl Thromb Hemost.* 2007;13(2):130-136.

18. Ulfman LH, Leusen JHW, Savelkoul HFJ, Warner JO, van Neerven RJJ. Effects of bovine immunoglobulins on immune function, allergy, and infection. *Front Nutr.* 2018; 5:52. http://dx.doi.org/10.3389/fnut.2018.00052
19. Olasehinde TA, Olaniran AO, Okoh AI. Therapeutic potentials of microalgae in the treatment of Alzheimer's disease. *Molecules.* 2017;22(3):480. http://dx.doi.org/10.3390/molecules22030480
20. Guan W et al. Co-morbidity and its impact on 1590 patients with COVID-19 in China: a nationwide analysis. *European Respiratory Journ*al 2020 55: 2000547; DOI: 10.1183/13993003.00547-2020
21. Steinbrenner H, Al-Quraishy S, Dkhil MA, Wunderlich F, Sies H. Dietary selenium in adjuvant therapy of viral and bacterial infections. *Adv Nutr.* 2015;6(1):73-82. http://dx.doi.org/10.3945/an.114.007575.73
22. Xiang D-X, Chen Q, Pang L, Zheng C-L. Inhibitory effects of silver nanoparticles on H1N1 influenza A virus in vitro. *J Virol Methods.* 2011;178(1-2):137-142. http://dx.doi.org/10.1016/j.jviromet.2011.09.003
23. Gaikwad S, Ingle A, Gade A, et al. Antiviral activity of mycosynthesized silver nanoparticles against herpes simplex virus and human parainfluenza virus type 3. *Int J Nanomedicine.* 2013; 8:4303-4314. http://dx.doi.org/10.2147/IJN.S50070

Chapter Twelve

1. Herington, Heather. *Transforming Trauma, a drugless and creative path to healing PTS.* Available 2021.

Chapter Thirteen

1. Neustadt J. Western Diet and Inflammation. *Integr Med.* 2006;5(4):14-18. https://todayspractitioner.com/wp-content/uploads/2014/04/0806_neustadt.pdf.
2. Pizzorno J. Glutathione! *Integr Med* (Encinitas). 2014;13(1):8-12.
3. Anderson RC, Anderson JH. Respiratory toxicity of mattress emissions in mice. *Arch Environ Health.* 2000;55(1):38-43. http://dx.doi.org/10.1080/00039890009603383
4. Landrigan PJ, Goldman LR. Children's vulnerability to toxic

chemicals: a challenge and opportunity to strengthen health and environmental policy. *Health Aff (Millwood)*. 2011;30(5):842-850. http://dx.doi.org/10.1377/hlthaff.2011.0151

5. Bruckner JV. Differences in sensitivity of children and adults to chemical toxicity: the NAS panel report. *Regul Toxicol Pharmacol*. 2000;31(3):280-285. http://dx.doi.org/10.1006/rtph.2000.1393
6. Mackowiak PA. Recycling metchnikoff: probiotics, the intestinal microbiome and the quest for long life. *Front Public Health*. 2013;1:52. http://dx.doi.org/10.3389/fpubh.2013.00052

Chapter Fourteen

1. Pizzorno J. Glutathione! *Integr Med (Encinitas)*. 2014;13(1):8-12.
2. Sanchez A, Reeser JL, Lau HS, et al. Role of sugars in human neutrophilic phagocytosis. *Am J Clin Nutr*. 1973;26(11):1180-1184.
3. Fahy JV, Dickey BF. Airway mucus function and dysfunction. *N Engl J Med*. 2010;363(23):2233-2247. http://dx.doi.org/10.1056/NEJMra0910061
4. Elderman M, Sovran B, Hugenholtz F, et al. The effect of age on the intestinal mucus thickness, microbiota composition and immunity in relation to sex in mice. *PLoS One*. 2017;12(9):e0184274. http://dx.doi.org/10.1371/journal.pone.0184274
5. Huang L, Szewczyk G, Sarna T, Hamblin MR. Potassium iodide potentiates broad-spectrum antimicrobial photodynamic inactivation using Photofrin. *ACS Infect Dis*. 2017;3(4):320-328. http://dx.doi.org/10.1021/acsinfecdis.7b00004
6. Zhao Y, Yu Y-B. Intestinal microbiota and chronic constipation. *Springerplus*. 2016;5(1):1130. http://dx.doi.org/10.1186/s40064-016-2821-1
7. Foster JA, Rinaman L, Cryan JF. Stress & the gut-brain axis: Regulation by the microbiome. *Neurobiol Stress*. 2017;7:124-136. http://dx.doi.org/10.1016/j.ynstr.2017.03.001
8. Pilch W, Pokora I, Szygu□a Z, et al. Effect of a single finnish sauna session on white blood cell profile and cortisol levels in athletes and non-athletes. *J Hum Kinet*. 2013;39(1):127-135. http://dx.doi.org/10.2478/hukin-2013-0075

Chapter Fifteen

1. Ueno K, Yamaura K, Nakamura T, Satoh T, Yano S. Acetaminophen-induced immunosuppression associated with hepatotoxicity in mice. *Res Commun Mol Pathol Pharmacol.* 2000;108(3-4):237-251.
2. Davidson NJ, Sowden JM, Fletcher J. Defective phagocytosis in insulin controlled diabetics: evidence for a reaction between glucose and opsonising proteins. *J Clin Pathol.* 1984;37(7):783-786. http://dx.doi.org/10.1136/jcp.37.7.783

Chapter Sixteen

1. Griffiths RD, Jones C. Recovery from intensive care. *BMJ.* 1999;319(7207):427-429. http://dx.doi.org/10.1136/bmj.319.7207.427
2. Landsverk G. 10 coronavirus symptoms you may not be aware of, from malaise and dizziness to digestive issues. Businessinsider.com. https://www.businessinsider.com/rare-uncommon-symptoms-of-covid-19-coronavirus-2020-3. Published March 31, 2020.
3. Samsel A, Seneff S. Glyphosate's suppression of cytochrome P450 enzymes and amino acid biosynthesis by the gut microbiome: Pathways to modern diseases. *Entropy (Basel).* 2013;15(12):1416-1463.

Final Word

1. Roser M, Ritchie H, Ortiz-Ospina E, Hasell J. Coronavirus Pandemic (COVID-19). Our World in Data. 2020. https://ourworldindata.org/coronavirus.
2. Feuerbacher A, Luckmann J, Boysen O, Zikeli S, Grethe H. Is Bhutan destined for 100% organic? Assessing the economy-wide effects of a large-scale conversion policy. *PLoS One.* 2018;13(6):e0199025. http://dx.doi.org/10.1371/journal.pone.0199025
3. Feuer W. US now has more coronavirus cases than either China

or Italy. CNBC. https://www.cnbc.com/2020/03/26/usa-now-has-more-coronavirus-cases-than-either-china-or-italy.html. Published March 26, 2020.

Appendix B

1. Smith EA, Malone RE. "everywhere the soldier will be": Wartime tobacco promotion in the US military. *Am J Public Health*. 2009;99(9):1595-1602. https://doi.org/10.2105/AJPH.2008.152983
2. Van Epps HL. Influenza: exposing the true killer. *J Exp Med*. 2006;203(4):803-803. https://doi.org/10.1084/jem.2034fta
3. Price WA. *Nutrition and Physical Degeneration. 8th ed*. Price-Pottenger Nutrition Foundation; 2008.
4. Carlsen MH, Halvorsen BL, Holte K, et al. The total antioxidant content of more than 3100 foods, beverages, spices, herbs and supplements used worldwide. *Nutr J*. 2010;9(1):3. doi:10.1186/1475-2891-9-3.
5. Whalen K a, McCullough ML, Flanders WD, Hartman TJ, Judd S, Bostick RM. Paleolithic and Mediterranean Diet Pattern Scores Are Inversely Associated with Biomarkers of Inflammation and Oxidative Balance in Adults. *J Nutr*. 2016;(12):1217-1226. doi:10.3945/jn.115.224048.
6. Pérez-Jiménez J, Elena Díaz-Rubio M, Saura-Calixto F. Contribution of Macromolecular Antioxidants to Dietary Antioxidant Capacity: A Study in the Spanish Mediterranean Diet. *Plant Foods Hum Nutr*. 2015;70(4):365-370. doi:10.1007/s11130-015-0513-6.
7. Vasquez A. Antiviral Nutrition: Against Colds, Flu, Herpes, AIDS, Hepatitis, Ebola, Dengue, and Autoimmunity: A Concept-Based and Evidence-Based Handbook and Research ... Practical Use (Inflammation Mastery Series). International College of Human Nutrition and Functional Medicine ICHNFM.ORG; 2014.
8. Alan R.. Gaby. *Nutritional Medicine*. Fritz Perlberg; 2011.
9. Benzie IFF. Evolution of dietary antioxidants. *Comp Biochem Physiol Part A Mol Integr Physiol*. 2003;136(1):113-126. doi:10.1016/S1095-6433(02)00368-9.

Appendix C

1. Calderón-Garcidueñas L, Solt AC, Henríquez-Roldán C, et al. Long-term air pollution exposure is associated with neuroinflammation, an altered innate immune response, disruption of the blood-brain barrier, ultrafine particulate deposition, and accumulation of amyloid beta-42 and alpha-synuclein in children and young adults. *Toxicol Pathol.* 2008;36(2):289-310. https://doi.org/10.1177/0192623307313011
2. Hanlon WW. *Pollution and Mortality in the 19th Century.* Cambridge, MA: National Bureau of Economic Research; 2015. https://doi.org/10.3386/w21647
3. Burt E, Orris P, Buchanan S. Scientific evidence of health effects from coal use in energy generation. Noharm-uscanada.org. https://noharm-uscanada.org/sites/default/files/documents-files/828/Health_Effects_Coal_Use_Energy_Generation.pdf.
4. Claus SP, Guillou H, Ellero-Simatos S. The gut microbiota: a major player in the toxicity of environmental pollutants? *NPJ Biofilms Microbiomes.* 2016;2(1):16003. https://doi.org/10.1038/npjbiofilms.2016.3
5. Jiang X-Q, Mei X-D, Feng D. Air pollution and chronic airway diseases: what should people know and do? *J Thorac Dis.* 2016;8(1):E31-40. https://doi.org/10.3978/j.issn.2072-1439.2015.11.50
6. Etzel RA, ed. *Pediatric Environmental Health.* American Academy of Pediatrics; 2012.
7. Curtis K. Casarett and Doulls *Toxicology: The Bacis Science of Poisons.* 8th ed.; 2013.
8. Vallero D. *Fundamentals of Air Pollution.* 5th ed. Elsevier; 2014.
9. Mercurio SD. *Understanding Toxicology A Biologica Approach.* Jones and Barlett Learning; 2017

ACKNOWLEDGMENTS

This book would never have been completed without my intrepid editor Avi Gross and formatters Jessica Moffitt and Max Mitchell. I am particularly grateful for Jess's cover design and Avi's back cover words. Thank you all from the bottom of my heart.

In deepest gratitude to Dr. Alec Pekler for his overall contributions and especially his exposé of dietary issues during the 1918-19 flu pandemic pertinent to the American soldier, and to Dr. Atousa Mahdavi for her thoughtfully bold preface.

To Stephanie Seneff PhD, for her invaluable insights into toxicity and illness and all the other podcast guests on *Dr. Heather Uncensored.* To Rick Kirschner ND, Mary Bove ND and Paul Anderson NMD for their generous contributions to the naturopathic profession. To Clement Lee NMD for his intravenous Vitamin C protocol, traditional naturopath Cathey Clack Painter for help with the essential oil section, and Claudia MacDonald and Dawn Overstreet for recipes.

To my Bastyr housemates, Sheila Dunn ND, Mary Minor ND and Lyn Patrick ND, who taught me so much over those years, and with great fondness to the Bastyr class of 1987, especially Marian Small ND who drove me to school every day so long ago.

For the loving support of my family—Avi, Rebecca, Phil, Oscar, Elliot, Harv, Grace, Hart, my 99 year old Aunt Isabelle, Amy, Barb and Florrie; the sweetest friends, Miriam, Marianna, Lynne, Atousa, Florence, all my Sears sistahs particularly Aileen, Phyllis, Marjorie and Helen, Max and Elliott, Veena, Dominique and Jade, Jeff, Murray, Susan, Laurie, Roberta, Idelina, Joanne, Darcey, Rivka, Janice and my neighbors here at Horace Heidt—who made it possible.

And finally, words don't cut it in terms of recognizing Avi's steadfast belief in the book and in me. In short, his astute perceptions and our deep love never cease to amaze.

Made in the USA
Monee, IL
16 September 2025

25805307R00163